Handbook of
Non-Motor Symptoms
in Parkinson's Disease

Handbook of Non-Motor Symptoms in Parkinson's Disease

K Ray Chaudhuri
Pablo Martinez-Martin
Per Odin
Angelo Antonini

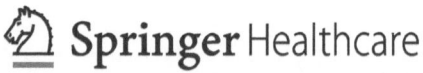

Published by Springer Healthcare Ltd, 236 Gray's Inn Road, London, WC1X 8HB, UK.

www.springerhealthcare.com

© 2011 Springer Healthcare, a part of Springer Science+Business Media.

British Library Cataloguing-in-Publication Data.

A catalogue record for this book is available from the British Library.

ISBN 978-1-907673-23-8

ISBN 978-1-908517-60-9 (eBook)

Project editor: Hannah Cole
Designer: Joe Harvey
Artworker: Sissan Mollerfors
Production: Marina Maher

Contents

Author biographies

K Ray Chaudhuri is a Consultant Neurologist and Professor in Neurology and Movement Disorders at King's College Hospital NHS Foundation Trust, University Hospital Lewisham, King's College London and the Institute of Psychiatry, London, UK. He is a recognized teacher and active researcher within the King's College London School of Medicine, London, and is the Medical Director of the National Parkinson Foundation International Centre of Excellence at King's College London. He also serves as Chairman of the RLS:UK group and of the International Parkinson's Disease Non-Motor Group, and is a member of the Movement Disorders Society appointments committee and the Task Force on Practice Parameters for Parkinson's disease and restless leg syndrome. For the Department of Health, UK, he serves on the steering group of the Medicines Management Committee and Gene Therapy Advisory Group, is an advisor of the Health Technology Assessment Committee, and is the lead clinician for the 18 week pathway for management of Parkinson's disease initiative. Prof. Chaudhuri is the author of 172 papers including reviews and book chapters, co-editor of four books on Parkinson's disease and restless legs syndrome (two in press), and has published over 150 peer-reviewed abstracts. He has contributed extensively to educational radio and television interviews, newspaper articles and videos. He has also lectured extensively on Parkinson's disease and restless legs syndrome at international meetings in Japan, continental Europe, India and Australia. His major research interests are drug treatment of Parkinson's disease and restless legs syndrome, parkinsonism in minority ethnic groups within the UK and abroad and sleep problems in Parkinson's disease. In 2005 he was awarded the DSc degree by the University of London and he received his personal Chair in Neurology in 2007.

Pablo Martinez-Martin, MD, PhD, is a neurologist and official researcher of the Spanish Public Boards of Research. Since 2006 he has been the

Scientific Director of the Research Unit for Alzheimer's disease, CIEN Foundation, at the Alzheimer Center Reina Sofia Foundation and a researcher at the Center for Biomedical Research in Neurodegenerative Diseases (CIBERNED). He has been a Researcher at the National Center for Epidemiology since 2007. All these three institutions belong to the Carlos III Institute of Health, Madrid, Spain. Between 1991 and 2001, Prof. Martinez-Martin was Head of the Department of Neurology at the University Hospital of Getafe, Madrid. He was Head of the Department of Neurology at the Central Hospital of the Red Cross, Madrid between 1989 and 1991 and Associate Professor of the Department of Medicine, Complutense University, Madrid between 1990 and 1994. Professor Martinez-Martin has been a member of the Movement Disorder Society Task Force for the revision of the Unified Parkinson's Disease Rating Scale (MDS-UPDRS) and other rating scales in Parkinson's disease since 2003. He was (2009–2011) a member of the National Institute of Neurological Disorders and Stroke (NINDS) Common Data Elements for Parkinson's Disease Working Group, Subgroup 'Scales and Statistics', the International Parkinson's Disease Non-Motor Symptoms Group, the EUROPAR group, and the SCales for Outcomes in PArkinson's disease (SCOPA) project. He is also a Principal Investigator for some international and Spanish nationwide studies and a member of the Official Spanish Registry for Human spongiform Encephalopathies. He has been a member, secretary, or chair of the Ethics Committee/IRB in the institutions where he has worked since 1990.

Prof. Martinez-Martin has received 12 awards in neurosciences, has published over 235 articles in scientific journals and has edited or co-edited 16 books. He is a member of the editorial boards for Movement Disorders, Parkinson's Disease, Neurología, and Revista de Neurología. His research interests are in patient assessment, patient-reported outcomes, caregiver's burden, health measures testing, and outcomes analysis, mainly applied to movement disorders and dementia.

Per Odin completed his medical education and received his PhD from the University of Uppsala, Sweden. Since 1987 his research and clinical studies have focused on movement disorders and he has held positions at the University of Lund, Sweden, the University School of Medicine, Hannover, Germany, and the University of Marburg, Germany.

Prof. Odin is currently Head of the Department of Neurology in Bremerhaven, Germany and has a research professorship at the University of Lund. His research interests are continuous dopaminergic stimulation, non-motor Parkinson's disease symptoms and cell replacement in Parkinson's disease. Prof. Odin is Chairman of the Swedish Parkinson Academy, and the Swedish and Scandinavian Movement Disorder Societies (SWEMODIS, ScandMODIS).

Angelo Antonini, MD, PhD, is Professor of Neurology and Director of the Parkinson Department at the Institute of Neurology IRCCS San Camillo in Venice. He earned his medical degree from the Università degli Studi di Roma 'La Sapienza', Rome. In November 1990 he completed his neurology training with honors and then undertook a visiting fellowship at the PET Department Paul Scherrer Institute, Villigen, Switzerland, before starting his PhD in neuroradiology under the supervision of Professor Klaus Leenders. In 1995 he received the first award from the National Parkinson Foundation for young researchers in Parkinson's disease. In 1996 he was awarded the Junior Faculty Award 1996/97 from United Parkinson Foundation and Parkinson's Disease Foundation for his research in the field of Parkinson's disease. From November 1997 to 2009 he worked at the Parkinson Institute in Milan where he coordinated clinical research at the Department of Neuroscience. His research focuses on pharmacology of dopaminergic medications and neuroimaging, as well as cognitive and behavioral aspects of Parkinson's disease. In addition he is actively involved in the use of continuous infusion of levodopa and apomorphine, as well as subthalamic nucleus deep brain stimulus (STN-DBS) for the treatment of motor fluctuations and dyskinesia of patients with complicated Parkinson's disease. During his academic career he has published over 200 peer-reviewed manuscripts and several book chapters. He serves as a reviewer for the main neurology journals and is on the editorial board of *Movement Disorders*.

Contributors

Kerstin Dietrich is a specialist in psychiatry and neurology currently in charge of the dementia subunit of the Department of Neurology in Bremerhaven, Germany.

Maria João Forjaz is a scientific researcher at the National School of Public Health, Spanish National Institute of Health Carlos III. She graduated from University of Lisbon, and she was a Fulbright scholar at University of North Texas, USA, where she obtained her doctorate in Clinical Psychology. She completed the clinical psychology internship at Rush University, Chicago. Her main research interests are quality of life in Parkinson's disease and older adults, assessment of non-motor symptoms, and scale validation using classic psychometric and Rasch analysis techniques. She is the principal investigator of several research grants on quality of life of older adults. Dr Forjaz is the author of nearly 30 articles in peer-review journal as well as several book chapters.

Monica Kurtis, MD, is a Consultant Neurologist and Director of the Movement Disorders Unit at the Hospital Ruber Internacional, Madrid, Spain. She obtained a BSc in Biological Science at the University of Edinburgh, Scotland and graduated from the Medical College of the Universidad de Navarra, Spain. She completed her residency in neurology at the Hospital Clínico San Carlos, Madrid, Spain and continued her training as a post doc clinical fellow in Movement Disorders at the College of Physicians and Surgeons at New York Presbyterian Hospital, Columbia University, USA. She has published numerous articles in peer reviewed journals and lectured on Parkinson's disease, other parkinsonisms, tics and dystonia. Her areas of interest include the impact of non-motor symptoms and medical/surgical treatment on quality of life in Parkinson's disease.

Kartik Logishetty graduated from Imperial College London, UK in surgery and anaesthesia. He is completing his medical training at King's College London before beginning an Academic Foundation post at the John Radcliffe Hospital, Oxford. He is a clinical research assistant in

Parkinson's disease, particularly focusing on the recognition and treatment of non-motor symptoms, at the National Parkinson Foundation Centre of Excellence at King's College Hospital, London.

Madhuja Tanya Mitra is currently completing her medical training at King's College London, UK. She graduated from King's College London with an intercalated BSc in neuroscience and neuropsychology and works as a clinical research assistant in Parkinson's disease focusing on non-motor symptoms at the National Parkinson Foundation Centre of Excellence at King's College Hospital, London. Upon graduating she will be undertaking an Academic Foundation Programme in Pediatrics.

Carmen Rodríguez-Blázquez is a psychologist currently working as a research assistant in the National Center of Epidemiology at the Carlos III Institute of Health, Madrid, Spain where she participates in several national and international research projects on the clinical and social aspects of neurological diseases (Parkinson's and Alzheimer's disease), the quality of life of older populations and the adaptation and validation of questionnaires. Previously, Carmen Rodríguez-Blázquez has worked as a co-researcher in projects on psychological disabilities and programs and services evaluation for the University of Cadiz, and the Universidad-Empresa of Cadiz, PROMI and Psicost Foundations, and as a Consultant for the Family and Social Affairs Office (Madrid Autonomous Community). She has co-authored several papers in indexed scientific journals and book chapters in the field of disabilities, neurological diseases, quality of life and the psychometric properties of scales and questionnaires.

Chandni Chandiramani graduated in India and completed a Neurosciences MSc at King's College London in 2010. She is a trained neuropsychologist and has an active interest in pursuing research addressing non-motor symptoms of Parkinson's disease.

Chapter 1

Introduction

Madhuja Tanya Mitra and K Ray Chaudhuri

The non-motor symptoms (NMSs) of Parkinson's disease (PD) remain an under-recognized and, consequently, under-treated set of symptoms. There is a wide variety of NMSs, ranging from neuropsychiatric and autonomic dysfunction to sleep disturbance and other symptoms. Figure 1.1 outlines the NMS complex of PD. Some NMSs can be related to dopaminergic treatment, such as dopamine dysregulation syndrome, drug-induced hallucinations or psychosis, and postural hypotension, whereas fluctuations in motor responses may also have major non-motor components – the so-called non-motor fluctuation [1]. In general, NMSs correlate with advancing disease [2], but some NMSs, such as rapid eye movement (REM) behavior disorder (RBD) and olfactory deficit, precede the onset of motor symptoms by a number of years. The pattern of various NMSs is, therefore, variable throughout the course of the disease.

Awareness of MNSs is integral to modern holistic care for PD, as some are potentially treatable and can enable significant improvements to health-related quality of life (HRQoL) of PD patients.

Pathophysiology of non-motor symptoms

Given the broad range of NMSs, their pathophysiology is complex and cannot be covered in detail here; additional detail can be found in the individual chapters. Broadly, the pathophysiological basis of NMSs in PD

K. R. Chaudhuri et al., *Handbook of Non-Motor Symptoms in Parkinson's Disease*, DOI: 10.1007/978-1-908517-60-9_1,
© Springer Healthcare, a part of Springer Science+Business Media 2011

can be subdivided into dopaminergic and non-dopaminergic. It is clear that some NMSs, such as hallucinations, dementia, postural hypotension, anxiety and sexual problems, have a relatively poor response to dopaminergic therapy whereas some are responsive to dopaminergic therapy

The spectrum of non-motor symptoms in Parkinson's disease
Neuropsychiatric symptoms
Depression
Anxiety
Apathy
Hallucinations, delusions, illusions
Delirium (may be drug induced)
Cognitive impairment (dementia, MCI)
Dopamine dysregulation syndrome (usually related to levodopa)
Impulse control disorders (related to dopaminergic drugs)
Panic attacks (could be 'off' related)
Sleep disorders and dysfunctions
REM sleep behavior disorder (possible pre-motor)
Excessive daytime somnolence, narcolepsy-type 'sleep attack'
Restless legs syndrome, periodic leg movements
Insomnia
Sleep-disordered breathing
NREM parasomnias (confusional wandering)
Fatigue
Central fatigue (may be related to dysautonomia)
Peripheral fatigue
Sensory symptoms
Pain (subtypes)
Olfactory disturbance
Hyposmia
Functional anosmia
Visual disturbance (blurred vision, diplopia), impaired contrast sensitivity
Autonomic dysfunction
Bladder urgency, frequency, nocturia
Sexual dysfunction (may be drug induced)
Sweating abnormalities (hyperhidrosis)
Orthostatic hypotension

Figure 1.1 The spectrum of non-motor symptoms in Parkinson's disease (continues opposite).

[3]. Central pathways including the serotoninergic and noradrenergic signaling are likely to be involved [4].

A novel concept of a six-stage pathological process of MNSs in PD was introduced by Braak and colleagues (Figure 1.2). Starting at induction sites with degeneration of the olfactory bulb and the anterior olfactory nucleus (clinically manifest as olfactory dysfunction) at stage 1, stage 2 reflects progression of the pathological process to the lower brain stem [5,6]. The

The spectrum of non-motor symptoms in Parkinson's disease (continued)
Gastrointestinal symptoms
Dribbling of saliva
Dysphagia
Ageusia
Constipation
Nausea
Vomiting
Reflux
Fecal incontinence
Dopaminergic drug-induced behavioral NMSs
Hallucinations, psychosis, delusions
Dopamine dysregulation syndrome (usually linked to levodopa intake)
Impulse control disorders (eg, compulsive gambling, hypersexuality, binge eating)
Dopaminergic drug-induced 'other' NMSs
Ankle swelling
Dyspnea (maybe linked to ergot dopamine agonist-related cardiac/respiratory failure)
Skin reactions
Subcutaneous nodules (apomorphine)
Erythematous rash (rotigotine patch)
Non-motor fluctuations
Dysautonomic
Cognitive/psychiatric
Sensory/pain
Visual blurring
Other symptoms
Weight loss
Weight gain (could be related to impulse control disorders)

Figure 1.1 The spectrum of non-motor symptoms in Parkinson's disease (continued). MCI, minimal cognitive impairment; NMS, non-motor symptom; NREM, non-rapid eye movement; REM, rapid eye movement.

lower brain stem involves several brain-stem nuclei, which are centers for mediating NMSs such as olfaction, sleep homeostasis, depression and cognition, pain, constipation, and central autonomic control.

This theory has popularized the concept of a 'bottom-up' pathogenesis of PD. In line with this theory, several NMSs of PD, such as hyposmia, RBD, constipation and depression, are now recognized as possible premotor features of PD (Figure 1.3).

The typical clinical motor triad, on which the current diagnosis of PD is based, emerges at Braak stages 3 and 4 with the involvement of the substantia nigra.

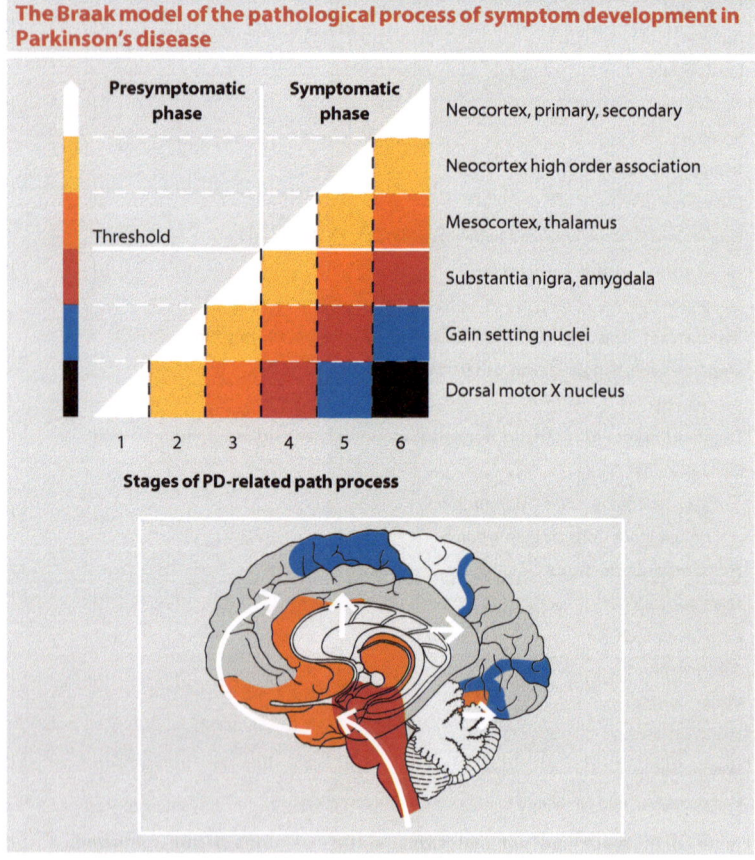

The Braak model of the pathological process of symptom development in Parkinson's disease

Figure 1.2 **The Braak model of the pathological process of symptom development in Parkinson's disease.** Adapted from [5].

Hawkes and Braak [7] have suggested a 'dual hit' hypothesis for pathogenesis of PD. An infective basis for PD has been proposed and it is postulated that a viral neurotropic agent may enter the brain via the nasal route, and undergo anterograde transmission by extensive existing connections of the olfactory bundle to the temporal lobe and other cortical areas, while a retrograde transmission may take place to the medulla via Meissner's plexus and vagal neurons.

Willis [8] has suggested that PD may be a neuroendocrine disorder, comprising a 'dopamine–melatonin' imbalance and involving the retinodiencephalo/mesencephalic–pineal axis. This appears to involve the visual system in the pathogenesis of PD in which vision is affected early.

The pattern of NMSs appears to be different, based on the stage of disease, and also perhaps reflects a progression of the underlying process as suggested by the Braak hypothesis. As such, cognitive problems usually dominate the late stage of PD [9]. However, the Braak staging is not without controversy because the concept relies on Lewy body deposition and not neuronal degeneration, and also does not fully

Non-motor symptoms suggested as preclinical (motor) characteristics in Parkinson's disease
Strong evidence
Constipation
Olfactory deficit
REM sleep behavior disorder
Depression
Suggested links (poor evidence base)
Restless legs syndrome
Apathy
Fatigue
Anxiety
Pain
Color vision
Erectile dysfunction
Excessive daytime sleepiness
Pre-morbid personality trait

Figure 1.3 Non-motor symptoms suggested as preclinical (motor) characteristics in Parkinson's disease.

explain why cognitive problems occur early, in, for example, dementia with Lewy bodies.

The burden of non-motor symptoms

A body of evidence suggests that the global burden of NMSs seems to have a greater impact on patients' quality of life (QoL) than their motor symptoms [10,11]. NMSs appear to affect HRQoL through a direct consequence of symptoms (eg depression and sleep dysfunction are determinants of HRQoL) and also indirectly, due to the disability caused by NMSs. Depression, poor sleep, dribbling of saliva, severe constipation, attention deficits and urinary problems can be severely detrimental to HRQoL [12,13]. These findings were echoed by a study demonstrating that the highest predictive value for poorer HRQoL was NMSs, including depression, sleep disorders and fatigue [14]. The same group found that depressive symptoms are common early in the disease, and have a substantial impact on patients' HRQoL, affecting many areas other than the obvious mental health dimension of the HRQoL profile [15].

NMSs cause a significant burden not only to the patient's life, but also to the caregiver's life. The caregiver's burden seems to be mostly affected by the patient's depression and impaired cognitive function, followed by sleep disturbances and hallucinations. A study specifically comparing the effect of motor and non-motor symptoms on the caregiver found that patient's depression and cognitive impairment had a greater impact on the caregiver's depression and strain than the patient's disability [16].

Finally, NMSs cause a large financial burden on the patient and the health-care system. NMSs such as falls, dementia and hallucinations are now recognized as some of the major reasons for admission to hospital and residential care [17,18]. Their hidden costs include loss of productivity of the patient and sometimes of the caregiver. Costs of advanced PD may be quadruple those of managing early PD, and are especially important to consider because the patient and often the spouse are elderly and may be living on a fixed pension or government benefits. Through early identification and treatment of NMSs, physicians will be able to provide PD patients with a better HRQoL, which will in turn limit the financial impact of PD [17,18]. It is also crucial that clinical trials of new therapies for PD include a focus on NMSs rather than the traditional approach of investigating motor symptoms only.

The burden of NMSs is discussed in detail in Chapter 2.

Recognizing and assessing non-motor symptoms
Challenges with recognizing non-motor symptoms

Despite the importance of recognizing NMSs in PD, studies have shown that clinicians often fail to identify them during consultations. This was first reported in a prospective study of 101 patients by Shulman and colleagues [19], who reported that neurologists failed to identify major NMSs such as depression, sleep disturbances, anxiety and fatigue in more than 50% of the patients. NMSs can easily be missed by the clinician because the consultation may solely focus on the motor aspect of the disease, the patient/caregiver does not mention the NMSs or the clinician fails to enquire about them [1]. Figure 1.4 provides a list of possible reasons as to why NMSs remain under recognized and under treated.

The PDLIFE study observed changes in self-reported health status of PD patients left untreated after diagnosis compared with patients on treatment [20]. It was found that the untreated group had worse health scores across all domains of the PD-specific PDQ-39 questionnaire (Parkinson's Disease Questionnaire – 39 items) compared with a group who were treated over an 18-month period [20]. The worsening of HRQoL appeared to be driven by deterioration of the several non-motor domains included in the PDQ-39 questionnaire. In many patients, it is likely that treatment was not started because clinicians relied on motor assessments alone, when there is also growing evidence that NMSs can be treatable.

A recent international study conducted by Chaudhuri et al [21] looked at the rates of non-declaration of NMSs to heath-care professionals. They collected data from 242 patients with PD across all age groups and stages attending outpatient clinics in specialist and elder-care settings. They used the Non-Motor Symptoms Questionnaire (NMSQuest), which is the first validated, self-completed, screening tool designed for rapid screening of NMSs, which contains 30 items across nine NMS domains and which empowers the patient and caregiver to flag up relevant NMSs

Possible explanations for poor recognition and treatment of non-motor symptoms

Lack of time for consultation in clinics

Focus on motor disorders in clinic

Lack of awareness of range of NMSs that can be associated with Parkinson's disease of:

- patients and caregivers
- doctors (Parkinson's disease nurse specialists are usually better informed in this area)

Embarrassment (of patients) to discuss some NMSs such as impulse control disorders, sexual problems, faecal incontinence

Perception of medical community that most NMSs are non-dopaminergic and untreatable

Perception of medical community that most NMSs are inevitable

Figure 1.4 Possible explanations for poor recognition and treatment of non-motor symptoms. NMS, non-motor symptoms.

that may not otherwise be discussed in consultations [22,23]. Patients were asked to fill in the questionnaire (with the aid of caregivers when necessary) in the waiting room before their consultation. After completion, patients were specifically asked if they had discussed the symptoms identified previously with any health-care professional and, if not, why not. Declaration of NMSs prompted appropriate review and management of individual symptoms in all patients [22].

This study discovered that NMSs are undisclosed in over 50% of cases. Delusions, daytime sleepiness, intense and vivid dreams, and dizziness were found to be the most frequently non-declared NMSs. When asked about why these were not declared, the patients and caregivers responded by outlining the following reasons:

- They were not aware that some of these symptoms may have been related to PD (delusions, RBD, intense and vivid dreams, pains, dribbling of saliva, insomnia).
- They were embarrassed to discuss these issues with the health-care professional unless they were prompted (sexual problems, incontinence of bowel).
- The consultation time was mostly occupied by discussion on motor symptoms and as such no or little time was available for discussion of any NMS-related issues [22].

The implication of this study is that, in more than 50% patients in this cohort, NMSs remained untreated despite treatment being available.

Tools for assessing non-motor symptoms

The under-recognition and non-disclosure of NMSs may be overcome by routinely using assessment scales in the clinical setting. Until 2006, no 'holistic' tools for either self-declaration or health-care professional-led detection of NMSs was available. The PD non-motor group led the development of the first tool designed to empower the patient and caregiver to declare NMSs in clinic; this is the NMSQuest, which is designed for completion while the patient awaits being seen. The NMSQuest has undergone extensive field validation and is a 30-item self-completed screening tool, with a 'yes/no' response format. It is endorsed by the Department of Health in the UK and is recommended for early use as a screening device for general practitioners to refer patients to secondary care; it is also recommended in the recently released SIGN (Scottish Intercollegiate Guidelines Network) guidelines from Scotland (January 2010) [24].

For scientific studies, clinical trials and clinic measurement of the effect of therapy in NMSs, the Non-Motor Symptoms Scale (NMSS) [25] is available and has been extensively validated in studies across Europe, Asia, the USA, Japan and South America, led by Martinez-Martin and Chaudhuri. The NMSS is a validated instrument that categorizes NMSs into 9 domains using 30 questions. The scale estimates the impact of NMSs by weighing each symptom by its frequency and severity, thus capturing the global burden for patients. Other available tools include the SCales for Outcomes in PArkinson's disease (SCOPA) battery of scales developed by van Hilten and colleagues from Leiden and the new version of the Unified Parkinson's Disease Rating Scale (UPDRS), the Movement Disorder Society (MDS)-UPDRS [26], which has a specific interview and questionnaire-led NMS section.

Assessment scales, including NMSQuest and NMSS, are discussed in greater detail in Chapters 3 and 4.

Treatment of non-motor symptoms

The importance of recognizing NMSs is underpinned by the fact that many NMSs of PD, contrary to common perception, are treatable and may respond to dopaminergic therapy [1]. The RECOVER study is the

Potentially treatable non-motor symptoms of Parkinson's disease undeclared to health-care professionals across several European centers

NMSs	Percentage undeclared	Potentially treatable using
Dribbling saliva	45.5	BTx, Atrovent spray, oral atropine, swallow timer
Vomiting	42.1	Domperidone
Constipation	46.1	Macrogol
Hallucinations	41.5	Relevant drug modifications/atypical neuroleptics
Anxiety	39.6	Anxiolytics
EDS	52.4	Modafinil, sleep hygiene, caffeine
RBD	44.1	Clonazepam, melatonin
Insomnia	43.9	Hypnotics, night-time CDD

Figure 1.5 Potentially treatable non-motor symptoms of Parkinson's disease undeclared to health-care professionals across several European centers. BTx, botulinum toxin injection; CDD, continuous drug delivery strategy. Adapted from [21].

A suggested scheme of clinical assessment of patients using non-motor tools, ensuring that holistic evaluation is undertaken

First clinical assessment of patient

NMSQuest completed by patient and caregiver

Clinical consultation with discussion of NMS flagged up in NMSQuest

Identification of NMS as treatable vs potentially untreatable and dopaminergic vs non-dopaminergic

Prioritize NMS according to prevalence and intrusiveness on day to day life/care

Treat highest-priority treatable symptom

Measure and monitor effect of treatment/intervention using NMSS

Figure 1.6 A suggested scheme of clinical assessment of patients using non-motor tools, ensuring that holistic evaluation is undertaken. NMS, non-motor symptom; NMSs, Non Motor Symptom Scale.

first double-blind, placebo-controlled study of a dopamine agonist that has used validated non-motor scales (PD Sleep Scale and NMSS) as primary and secondary outcome measures, showing a robust effect of dopaminergic therapy on aspects of sleep, which manifested as improvement in early morning states, pain and overall HRQoL [27].

Non-dopaminergic therapies remain the mainstay of NMS treatment. The American Academy of Neurology task force has extensively reviewed and provided evidence-based guidelines for the treatment of NMSs in PD [28]. Figure 1.5 provides a list of potentially treatable NMSs and their management. Despite the advances in management of PD, the evidence base for NMS treatment remains inadequate. There is a lack of controlled drug trials for the treatment of many NMSs including nocturia and apathy, and the evidence available is limited and contradictory. Therefore there must be a concerted effort to recognize NMSs and their management. Use of NMSQuest is highly recommended because this is a unique, clinimetrically validated tool that can flag NMSs and empower patients with PD. A suggested scheme for clinical assessment of patients, ensuring that relevant NMS are taken into consideration, is shown in Figure 1.6.

Management of the individual NMSs is discussed in Chapters 5–11.

References

1 Chaudhuri KR, Healy DG, Schapira AH. Non-motor symptoms of Parkinson's disease: diagnosis and management. *Lancet Neurol* 2006;5:235-245.

2 Martinez-Martin P, Schapira AH, Stocchi F, et al. Prevalence of nonmotor symptoms in Parkinson's disease in an international setting; study using nonmotor symptoms questionnaire in 545 patients. *Mov Disord* 2007;22:1623-1629.

3 Chaudhuri KR, Schapira AHV. The non motor symptoms of Parkinson's disease: dopaminergic pathophysiology and treatment. *Lancet Neurol* 2009;8:464-474.

4 Zgaljardic DJ, Foldi NS, Borod JC. Cognitive and behavioral dysfunction in Parkinson's disease: neurochemical and clinicopathological contributions. *J Neural Transm* 2004;111:1287-1301.

5 Braak H, Del Tredici K, Rüb U, et al. Staging of brain pathology related to sporadic Parkinson's disease. *Neurobiol Aging* 2003;24:197-211.

6 Del Tredici K, Braak H. Idiopathic Parkinson's disease: staging an α-synucleinopathy with a predictable pathoanatomy. In: Kahle P, Haass C (eds), Molecular Mechanisms in Parkinson's Disease. Georgetown, TX: Landes Bioscience, 2004:1-32.

7 Hawkes C, Del Tredici K, Braak H. Parkinson's disease: a dual hit hypothesis. *Neuropath Appl Neurobiol* 2007;33:599-614.

8 Willis GL. Parkinson's disease as a neuro-endocrine disorder of circadian function: dopamine melatonin imbalance and the visual system in the genesis and progression of the degenerative process. *Rev Neurosci* 2008;19:245-316.

9 Hely MA, Reid WG, Adena MA, et al. The Sydney multicenter study of Parkinson's disease: the inevitability of dementia at 20 years. *Mov Disord* 2008;23:837-844.

10 Global Parkinson's Disease Survey Steering Committee. Factors impacting on quality of life in Parkinson's disease: results from an international survey. *Mov Disord* 2002;17:60-67.

11 Lohle M, Storch A, Reichmann H. Beyond tremor and rigidity: non-motor features of Parkinson's disease. *J Neural Transm* 2009;116:1483-1492.

12 Chaudhuri K, Martinez-Martin P, Brown R. The metric properties of a novel non-motor symptoms scale for Parkinson's disease: Results from an international pilot study. *Mov Disord* 2007;22:1901-1911.

13 Martinez-Martin P, Rodriguez-Blazquez C, Abe K, et al. International study on the psychometric attributes of the non-motor symptoms scale in Parkinson disease. *Neurology* 2009;73:1584-1591.

14 Qin Z, Zhang L, Sun F, et al. Health related quality of life in early Parkinson's disease: impact of motor and non-motor symptoms, results from Chinese levodopa exposed cohort. *Parkinsonism Relat Disord* 2009;15:767-771.

15 Qin Z, Zhang L, Sun F, et al. Depressive symptoms impacting on health-related quality of life in early Parkinson's disease: results from Chinese l-dopa exposed cohort. *Clin Neurol Neurosurg* 2009b;111:733-737.

16 Carter JH, Stewart BJ, Lyons KS, Archbold PG. Do motor and nonmotor symptoms in PD patients predict caregiver strain and depression? *Mov Disord* 2008;23:1211-1216.

17 Keranen T, Kaakkola S, Sotaniemi K, et al. Economic burden and quality of life impairment increase with severity of PD. *Parkinsonism Relat Disord* 2003;9:163-168.

18 Chaudhuri KR, Yates L, Martinez-Martin P. The non-motor symptom complex of Parkinson's disease: a comprehensive assessment is essential. *Curr Neurol Neurosci Rep* 2005;5:275-283.

19 Shulman LM, Taback RL, Rabinstein AA, Weiner WJ. Non-recognition of depression and other non-motor symptoms in Parkinson's disease. *Parkinsonism Relat Disord* 2002;8:193-197.

20 Grosset D, Taurah L, Burn DJ, et al. A multicentre longitudinal observational study of changes in self reported health status in people with Parkinson's disease left untreated at diagnosis. *J Neurol Neurosurg Psychiatry* 2007;78:465-469.

21 Chaudhuri KR, Prieto-Jurcynska C, Naidu Y, et al. The nondeclaration of nonmotor symptoms of Parkinson's disease to health care professionals: an international study using the nonmotor symptoms questionnaire. *Mov Disord* 2010;25:697-701.

22 Chaudhuri KR, Martinez-Martin P, Schapira AH, et al. International multicenter pilot study of the first comprehensive self-completed nonmotor symptoms questionnaire for Parkinson's disease: the NMSQuest study. *Mov Disord* 2006;21: 916-923.

23 Chaudhuri KR, Martinez-Martin P. Quantitation of non-motor symptoms in Parkinson's disease. *Eur J Neurol* 2008;15(suppl 2):2-7.

24 Scottish Intercollegiate Guidelines Network. Diagnosis and pharmacological management of Parkinson's disease. Available online at www.sign.ac.uk/pdf/sign113.pdf. Last accessed August 2011.

25 Chaudhuri KR, Martinez-Martin P, Brown RG, et al. The metric properties of a novel non-motor symptoms scale for Parkinson's disease: Results from an international pilot study. *Mov Disord* 2007;22:1901-1911.

26 Goetz CG, Tilley BC, Shaftman SR, et al. Movement Disorder Society-sponsored revision of the Unified Parkinson's Disease Rating Scale (MDS-UPDRS): scale presentation and clinimetric testing results. *Mov Disord* 2008;23:2129-2170.

27 Trenkwalder C, Chaudhuri K, Anderson TB, et al; for the RECOVER Study Group. Effect of rotigotine on control of early morning motor function and sleep quality in subjects with idiopathic Parkinson's disease. *Parkinsonism Relat Disord* 2009;15(suppl 136):2.170.

28 Zesiewicz TA, Sullivan KL, Arnulf I, et al. Practice parameter: treatment of nonmotor symptoms of Parkinson disease: report of the Quality Standards Subcommittee of the American Academy of Neurology. *Neurology* 2010;74:924-931.

Chapter 2

The burden of non-motor symptoms

Maria João Forjaz, Chandni Chandiramani and
Pablo Martinez-Martin

Although most of the symptoms of Parkinson's disease (PD) seem to
be motor-based, the non-motor symptoms (NMSs) of PD, often over-
shadowed, also constitute a major clinical challenge. The NMSs of PD,
including neuropsychiatric, cognitive, gastrointestinal and sensory,
not only are observed in later stages but also predominate in the early
stages of PD. Research suggests that NMSs are present at onset, while
some can precede the motor symptoms, often by many years [1–3]. The
identification of premotor stages is based on the early detection of the
combination of NMSs with PD detection: for example, olfactory changes
are the most common NMS presenting in the early stages of PD and occur
in 90% of the patients [4,5]. Surveys reveal that 90% have at least one
NMS, whereas 10% of PD patients exhibit five NMSs [6]. NMSs seem
to be present before the diagnosis of PD and also inevitably emerge
with progression of the disease, thus having an impact on patients'
health-related quality of life (HRQoL) and placing an increased burden
on caregivers.

K. R. Chaudhuri et al., *Handbook of Non-Motor Symptoms
in Parkinson's Disease*, DOI: 10.1007/978-1-908517-60-9_2,
© Springer Healthcare, a part of Springer Science+Business Media 2011

The burden of non-motor symptoms on patients' health-related quality of life

Two important shifts

Interest in patients' HRQoL, and patient-reported outcomes including QoL measures, started when therapeutic interventions changed their focus from postponing death to improving HRQoL. As PD is a chronic debilitating condition, so far without cure, specialists became interested in measuring the impact of the disease and treatments in terms of HRQoL [7,8].

Recently, a second shift occurred, and there has been growing interest in measuring not only motor symptoms, but also NMSs. First, measures about specific NMSs, developed for the general population, were included in PD studies. Later on, there was an effort to develop domain-specific questionnaires for PD, such as the SCales for Outcomes in PArkinson's disease (SCOPA). Finally, specific scales, comprising a large number of NMSs in a single measure, such as the NMS Questionnaire (NMSQuest) and the NMS Scale (NMSS), were developed [9].

Studies using non-motor symptom measures

There is a high consistency of findings in studies using PD-specific NMS measures (Figure 2.1). Patients report, on average, 9–11 symptoms on the NMSQuest, the most frequent symptoms being nocturia, urgency, constipation and 'the blues'. The number of symptoms increases with Hoehn and Yahr (H&Y) stage [22] and disease duration. The mean severity score on the NMSS ranges from 31 to 91.

The most common NMSS domains are mood and sleep, and the NMSS scores are significantly associated with H&Y stage and motor symptoms. The relationship between NMSS and HRQoL is high, consistent and robust (Spearman $r = 0.70$ with PDQ-39 or -8) [15,18].

Motor versus non-motor symptoms: effect on patients' health-related quality of life

NMSs seem to have a greater impact on patients' HRQoL than motor symptoms [23–25]. The most frequent HRQoL determinants found in a HRQoL review of PD were depression and H&Y stage, followed by disability, disease duration and gait disorders [7].

A study specifically analyzing the impact of motor symptoms and NMSs on patients' HRQoL found that, although motor variables contributed to 19% of the variance, inclusion of non-motor factors significantly improved the model (62%) [26]. The most important predictors of HRQoL were depression, sleep disorders and fatigue and, to a lesser extent, UPDRS motor score and H&Y stage.

Further research

NMSs have a great impact on patients' HRQoL. This relationship, when using the NMSS, is robust and of high magnitude. More research is needed to ascertain which domains of the NMSS mostly impact on which HRQoL aspects, and whether NMSs predict HRQoL in the medium or long term. Longitudinal studies are very important, because there is strong evidence that some NMSs may be preclinical characteristics of PD [27]. Finally, there are insufficient studies comparing the contribution of motor and non-motor symptoms on HRQoL, using specific NMS measures.

The burden of patient's non-motor symptoms on the caregiver

NMSs cause a significant burden to not only the patient's life, but also the caregiver's life. Figure 2.2 summarizes the main studies about the patient factors influencing the caregiver's QoL and burden.

The impact of the disease on the caregiver's wellbeing can be measured in terms of QoL or specific measures of burden. Questionnaires of the caregiver's QoL include the SF-36 [52], EQ-5D [53], WHOQOL-BREF [54] and the Scale of Quality of Life of Caregivers [55]. Older patients with lower HRQoL, higher disability and more severe motor and neuropsychological affectation are taken care of by caregivers with lower HRQoL [37,39,45,49].

There are several measures of caregivers' burden, the three most commonly used measures being: the Zarit Caregiver Burden Inventory [56]; the Caregiver Burden Inventory [57]; and the Subjective and Objective

Studies using specific non-motor symptom scales for Parkinson's disease

Reference	Sample	Symptoms, domains or score: M ± SD (range)	Most common symptoms or domains	Associated factors
NMSQuest	**n = 100–545**	**Mean number of symptoms: 9 to 11**	**Nocturia, urgency, constipation, depression**	**H&Y stage, disease duration**
Chaudhuri, et al (2006) [10]	123 PD patients (multinational)	Symptoms: 9.6	Symptoms: nocturia (67%), urgency (61%), remembering (51%)	H&Y stage (r = 0.31), disease duration (r = 0.22)
Martinez-Martin, et al (2007) [11]	545 PD patients (multinational)	Symptoms: 10.3 ± 5.4 (0–28)	Symptoms: nocturia (62%), urgency (56%), constipation (52%) Domains: digestive, sleep	Age of onset (before/after 50 years), disease duration, H&Y stage
Chaudhuri, et al (2010) [12]	242 PD patients (multinational)	Symptoms: 10.9 ± 5.6	Symptoms: nocturia (65%), urgency (60%), concentrating (50%) Domains: gastrointestinal, sleep	NMSs present more in akinesia PD type
Wang, et al (2010) [13]	117 PD patients (China)	Not reported	Symptoms: constipation (56%), sad/blues (43%), remembering (41%)	Malnutrition
Cervantes-Arriaga, et al (2010) [14]	100 PD patients (Mexico)	Symptoms: 10.6 ± 5.5 (1–26)	Not reported	H&Y (r <0.25, p <0.05)
NMSS	**n = 22–242**	**Mean of NMSS scores: 31–90**	**Domains: mood and sleep**	**H&Y stage, quality of life, motor symptoms**
Chaudhuri, et al (2007) [15]	242 PD patients (multinational)	NMSS score: 56.5 ± 40.7 (0–243)	Not reported	PDQ-8 (r = 0.70); H&Y (r = 0.33); UPDRS section 4 (r = 0.49); UPDRS section 3 (r = 0.35)
Honig, et al (2009) [16]	22 patients with advanced PD receiving intrajejunal levodopa infusion (multinational)	NMSS score at baseline: 89.9 ± 56.5; at follow-up: 39.4 ± 33.9	Not reported	Change in NMSS score associated with: PDQ-8 (r = 0.61). UPDRS complications (r = 0.55); dyskinesia score (r = 0.41) and proportion of day in off (r = 0.54)

		Number of symptoms	Symptoms / Domains	Correlations
Kim, et al (2009) [17]	23 new PD patients (Korea)	Number of symptoms: 8.3 ±4.0 (3–17). NMSS score: 37.0 ±28.9	Symptoms: nocturia (65%), forget things (61%), restless legs (52%)	H&Y stage (r = 0.43, with number of symptoms)
Martinez-Martin, et al (2009) [18]	411 PD patients (multinational)	NMSS score: 57.1 ±44.0 (0–233)	Domains with higher mean scores: mood/apathy (11.2), sleep/fatigue (9.6), urinary (9.0)	Group differences: disease duration, H&Y stage and CISI-PD severity level (p <0.001). Correlations: PDQ-39 (r = 0.70). SCOPA-AUT (r = 0.64). EQ-5D index (r = 0.57). Other correlations (r = 0.38–0.51): H&Y: SCOPA-M, -PC and -COG; CISI-PD; PDSS
Wang, et al (2009) [19]	126 PD patients (China)	NMSS score: 31.06 ± 30.88 (0–177)	Domains with higher mean scores: mood (8.26), sleep/fatigue (6.33), miscellany (3.84)	Correlations with: sleep (PSQI, r = 0.63); anxiety (HAMA, r = 0.52); depression (GDS, r = 0.45)
Cervantes-Arriaga, et al (2010) [14]	100 PD patients (Mexico)	NMSS score: 69.7 ±56.9 (0–237)	Not reported	H&Y (r < 0.25, p 0.05)
Checklist of 48 NMSs grouped into 12 domains	**n = 1072–1130**	**Mean number of symptoms: 8**	**Domains: gastrointestinal**	**H&Y stage, quality of life**
Barone, et al (2009) [20]	1072 PD patients (Italy)	Symptoms: 7.8 ±4.9 (0–32) Domains: 5.5 ±2.5 (0–12)	Symptoms: fatigue (58%), anxiety (56%), leg pain (38%) Domains: psychiatric (67%), sleep (64%), gastrointestinal (61%)	H&Y stage (all domains except cardiovascular); cognitive impairment (6 domains); PDQ-39 (all domains)
Colosimo, et al (2010) [21]	1130 PD patients (Italy)	Symptoms: 8 Domains: 5.5	Domains: gastrointestinal (62%), pain (61%), urinary (58%)	None analyzed

Figure 2.1 Studies using specific non-motor symptom scales for Parkinson's disease. CISI-PD, Clinical Impression of Severity Index for Parkinson's Disease; GDS, Geriatric Depression Scale; HAMA, Hamilton Rating Scale for Anxiety; H&Y, Hoehn and Yahr scale; NMS, non-motor symptom; NMSQuest, Non-Motor Symptoms Questionnaire; NMSS, Non-Motor Symptoms Scale; PD, Parkinson's disease; PDQ-39, Parkinson's disease Questionnaire – 39 items; PDQ-8, Parkinson's disease Questionnaire – 8 items; SCOPA-AUT, SCales for Outcomes in PArkinson's disease – Autonomic; SCOPA-COG, SCales for Outcomes in PArkinson's disease – Cognition; SCOPA-M, SCales for Outcomes in PArkinson's disease – Motor; SCOPA-PC, SCales for Outcomes in PArkinson's Disease – Psychiatric Complications; UPDRS, Unified Parkinson's disease Rating Scale.

Studies about patient's factors influencing the caregiver's quality of life

Reference	Study type: sample, country, design	Patient factors: disease related, NMS, motor symptoms, others	Outcome measure: caregiver's burden; caregiver's QoL
Miller et al (1998) [28]	54 dyads (patient–caregiver), UK, multiple regression	**NMS:** depression	**Caregiver's burden:** GHQ-30, Depression (GDS, BDI); Machine Strain Scale
Carter et al (2004) [29]	380 caregivers, USA, group differences	**Disease related:** disease severity	**Caregiver's burden:** Family Care(giving) Inventory
Meara et al (1999) [30]	79 caregivers, UK, correlations	**NMS:** depression, cognition **Disease related:** disease severity	**Caregiver's burden:** depression (GDS-15)
Habermann (2000) [31]	8 caregivers, USA, qualitative study	**NMS:** Feelings of struggle and frustration	**Caregiver's burden:** interview about challenges that CG experience
Fernandez et al (2001) [32]	45 dyads, USA, multiple regression	**Disease related:** disease duration	**Caregiver's burden:** depression (HAMD, BDI)
Caap-Ahlgren and Dehlin (2002) [33]	65 dyads, Sweden, multiple regression	**NMS:** depression **Others:** disability	**Caregiver's burden:** scale, depression (GDS)
Edwards and Scheetz (2002) [34]	41 caregivers, USA, multiple regression	**Others:** activities of daily living	**Caregiver's burden:** Zarit Caregiver Burden Inventory
Happe and Berger (2002) [35]	106 caregivers, Germany, multiple regression	**Disease related:** disease severity (with caregiver's sleep) **NMS:** depression (with caregiver's depression), sleep (with caregiver's sleep)	**Caregiver's burden:** Caregiver Burden Inventory, depression (CES-D); sleep
Thommessen et al (2002) [36]	58 couples, Norway, structural equation modelling	**NMS:** cognition, depression	**Caregiver's burden:** Relative Stress Scale

Martinez-Martin et al (2004) [37]	86 dyads, Spain, correlations	**Disease related:** disease duration and severity **NMS:** Neuropsychological disorders Questionnaire (verbal communication, mental state, depression, sleep, bladder incontinence, perception alterations) **Motor symptoms:** UPDRS (I–IV) **Others:** disability	**Caregiver's QoL:** Scale of Quality of Life of Caregivers
Pal et al (2004) [38]	40 PD patients and 23 caregivers, Canada, correlations	**NMS:** depression, anxiety and sleep	**Caregiver's burden:** caregiver's depression, anxiety and sleep
Martinez-Martin et al (2005) [39]	57 dyads, Spain, multiple regression	**Motor symptoms:** UPDRS (I–III) **Others:** disability (ISAPD-ADL); QoL (PDQ-8)	**Caregiver's QoL:** Scale of Quality of Life of Caregivers
Cifu et al (2006) [40]	49 dyads, USA, correlations	**Disease related:** disease severity **NMS:** cognition **Motor symptoms:** motor examination **Others:** disability	**Caregiver's burden:** Zarit Caregiver Burden Inventory; Caregiver Distress Scale
Schrag et al (2006) [41]	123 caregivers, UK, correlations	**Disease related:** disease duration and severity **NMS:** depression, hallucinations, confusion, falls **Others:** disability, QoL	**Caregiver's burden:** Caregiver Burden Inventory, depression (BDI) **Caregiver's QoL:** Scale of Quality of life of Caregivers
Schestatsky et al (2006) [42]	21 dyads, Brazil, correlations	**Others:** patient's age	**Caregiver's QoL:** WHOQOL-BREF

Figure 2.2 Studies about patient's factors influencing the caregiver's quality of life (continues overleaf).

Studies about patient's factors influencing the caregiver's quality of life (continued)

Reference	Study type: sample, country, design	Patient factors: disease related, NMS, motor symptoms, others	Outcome measure: caregiver's burden; caregiver's QoL
Aarsland et al (2007) [43]	94 caregivers, Norway, multiple regression	**NMS:** depression, cognition (Relative Stress Scale), depression, neuropsychiatric symptoms, cognition (caregiver's depression and distress)	**Caregiver's burden:** Relative Stress Scale; depression (BDI); distress (GHQ-12)
Aarsland et al (2007) [43]	537, multinational, descriptive	**NMS:** agitation, psychosis, mood	**Caregiver's burden:** caregiver's distress (Neuropsychiatric Inventory)
Kim et al (2007) [44]	76 caregivers, Korea, group differences	**Disease related:** disease duration (with subjective burden) and severity (with objective burden); **Others:** disability (UPDRS II with objective and subjective burden)	**Caregiver's burden:** subjective and objective Burden Scale
Martinez-Martin et al (2007) [45]	80 dyads, Spain, multiple regression	**Disease related:** disease severity; **NMS:** mood (depression, anxiety); **Others:** QoL (EQ-5D), disability	**Caregiver's burden:** Zarit Caregiver Burden Inventory, HADS; **Caregiver's QoL:** SF-36, EQ-5D
Carter et al (2008) [46]	219 caregivers, USA, multiple regression	**Disease related:** cognition (delayed recall), depression; **Others:** disability (UPDRS-ADL)	**Caregiver's burden:** Family Care (giving) Inventory; depression (CES-D)
Lokk (2008) [47]	404 caregivers, Sweden, structured interview	**Disease related:** disease duration; **NMS:** cognition, hallucinations, memory, bradyphrenia, sleep; **Motor symptoms:** motor dysfunction, motor complications	**Caregiver's burden:** questions about perceived worry, stress, mood and sleep; **Caregiver's QoL:** EQ-5D visual analogue scale (0–10)

Study	Sample	Factors	Caregiver's burden / QoL
Martinez-Martin et al (2008) [48]	286 dyads, Spain, multiple regression	**Disease related:** disease severity (with caregiver's burden and depression) **NMS:** sleep, cognition, NMS (with caregiver's burden), NMS (with caregiver's QoL) **Motor symptoms:** motor complications (with caregiver's burden) **Others:** disability, QoL, age (with caregiver's burden), patient's QoL (with caregiver's QoL)	**Caregiver's burden:** Zarit Caregiver Burden Inventory, caregiver's anxiety and depression (HADS) **Caregiver's QoL:** EQ-5D
D'Amelio et al (2009) [49]	Caregivers, Italy, path analysis	**NMS:** behavioral problems (with burden); cognitive impairment (with QoL) **Others:** patient–caregiver relationship (with burden); perceived social support (with burden); frequency of breaks (with QoL)	**Caregiver's burden:** Caregiver Burden Inventory **Caregiver's QoL:** Scale of Quality of Life of Caregivers
Stella et al (2009) [50]	50 dyads, Brazil, correlations	**Disease related:** disease severity and age of onset (dementia group) **NMS:** neuropsychiatric symptoms **Others:** UPDRS functional (dementia and depression patient groups)	**Caregiver's burden:** distress score of Neuropsychiatric Inventory
Roland et al (2010) [51]	5 spouses, Canada, semi-qualitative	**Others:** motor fluctuations, safety	**Caregiver's burden:** repertory grid

Figure 2.2 Studies about patient's factors influencing the caregiver's quality of life (continued). BDI, Beck Depression Inventory; CES-D, Center for Epidemiologic Studies Depression Scale; GDS, Geriatric Depression Scale; GHQ2, General Health Questionnaire-2; HADS, Hospital Anxiety and Depression Scale; HAMD, Hamilton Rating Scale for Depression; H&Y, Hoehn and Yahr staging; ISAPD, Intermediate Scale for Assessment of Parkinson's Disease; NMS, non-motor symptoms; PD, Parkinson's disease; PDQ-8, Parkinson's disease Questionnaire – 8 items; QoL, quality of life; SF-36, Short Form Health Survey – 36 items; UPDRS, Unifies Parkinson's Disease Rating Scale; WHOQOL-BREF, World Health Organization Quality of Life – Brief.

Burden Scale [58]. Measures of specific symptoms or general distress have also been used to measure caregivers' burden.

The disease-related factors that most affect caregivers' burden are severity and duration. Almost half of the revised studies identified the patient's disability as an important determinant of the caregiver's burden. However, few studies found a significant association between motor dysfunction and the caregiver's burden [37,40,47,48]. Relative to NMSs, the caregiver's burden seems to be mostly affected by the patient's depression and impaired cognitive function, followed by sleep disturbances and hallucinations. A study specifically comparing the effect of motor and non-motor symptoms in the caregiver found that a patient's depression and cognitive impairment had a greater impact on a caregiver's depression and strain than a patient's disability [46]. Research about the impact of NMSs, using specific NMS measures, on caregivers' burdens and QoL is needed.

Economic costs

PD is the second most common neurodegenerative disorder; it increases with age and affects about 1 million people in the USA and about 5 million people worldwide [59]. Given the progressive nature of PD, such an increase will have a significant impact on the burden of the health-care system and caregivers, with considerable caregiving required in the later stages of PD [59].

NMSs range from autonomic and neuropsychiatric symptoms to sleep disturbances and sensory problems. Although cognitive impairment has a lesser impact compared with other NMSs, it continues to be one of the major reasons for admission to institutional care [60,61]. Autonomic dysfunction can occur early in the disease and may not necessarily be related to disease severity. One study reported that half the sample of hospitalized PD patients rated autonomic symptoms as 'a lot' or 'very much' [62].

In the UK, the annual direct costs for patients living in full-time institutional care was estimated at about £19 338, five times higher than in the home setting [63]. Costs for NMS drug therapy increase with clinical progression of symptoms, thus contributing to higher economic costs, especially for patients with a fixed income from pensions and government benefits [61,64]. Economic costs are doubled by each H&Y stage, especially after stage 2.0 [65].

NMSs also account for the burden of hidden costs such as sick leave, early retirement and informal care not only for patients but also for caregivers in certain instances. The cost burden of NMSs is significantly high, especially in patients with advanced PD and increasingly severe symptoms, for whom there is a poorer QoL, reduced productivity and a greater need for health-care services, which in turn have an impact on direct and indirect costs.

Thus, identifying disease-modifying treatments early in the disease, before any functional or motor disability appears, is critical in reducing costs and preserving QoL. Evidence suggests that initial therapy with non-levodopa agents is cost-effective, prolongs time to levodopa initiation and delays the onset of dyskinesias [66,67]. Results of the ADAGIO trial hint that rasagiline can reduce the progression of NMSs, as assessed using Movement Disorder Society (MDS)-UPDRS [68–70].

Conclusions

There is a significant interrelationship of severity of disease, QoL, patient's and caregiver's burden, and cost of illness. NMSs contribute to the overall PD burden, which is a major determinant of QoL. An increasing awareness of 'at-risk' individuals, based on detection of some or a combination of NMSs, is essential for an early identification of PD patients. Identification of prodromal patients plays a key factor in preventing the burden of economic costs and improving QoL of patients and caregivers. Keeping this in mind, it becomes important to optimize the management of all aspects of NMSs in PD.

References

1   Shiba M, Bower JH, Maraganore DM, et al. Anxiety disorders and depressive disorders preceding Parkinson's disease: a case-control study. *Mov Disord* 2000;15:669-677.
2   Iranzo A, Molinuevo JL, Santamaria J, et al. Rapid-eye-movement sleep behavior disorder as an early marker for a neurodegenerative disorder: a descriptive study. *Lancet Neurol* 2006;5:572-577.
3   Antonini A. Non-motor symptoms in Parkinson's disease. *Eur Neurol Rev* 2009;4:25-27.
4   Mueller A, Abolmaali ND, Hakimi AR, et al. Olfactory bulb volumes in patients with idiopathic Parkinson's disease a pilot study. *J Neural Transm* 2005;112:1363-1370.
5   Berendse HW. I. 4 Early diagnosis in PD: olfaction. *Parkinsonism Rel Disord* 2006;12:1-2.

6 Miyasaki JM, Shannon K, Voon V, et al. Practice Parameter: evaluation and treatment of depression, psychosis, and dementia in Parkinson disease (an evidence-based review): report of the Quality Standards Subcommittee of the American Academy of Neurology. *Neurology* 2006;66:996-1002.

7 Forjaz MJ, Frades-Payo B, Martinez-Martin P. [The current state of the art concerning quality of life in Parkinson's disease: II. Determining and associated factors.] *Rev Neurol* 2009;49:655-660.

8 Frades-Payo B, Forjaz MJ, Martinez-Martin P. [The current state of the art concerning quality of life in Parkinson's disease: I. Instruments, comparative studies and treatments]. *Rev Neurol* 2009;49:594-598.

9 Chaudhuri KR, Martinez-Martin P. Quantitation of non-motor symptoms in Parkinson's disease. *Eur J Neurol* 2008;15(suppl 2):2-7.

10 Chaudhuri KR, Martinez-Martin P, Schapira AH, et al. International multicenter pilot study of the first comprehensive self-completed nonmotor symptoms questionnaire for Parkinson's disease: the NMSQuest study. *Mov Disord* 2006;21:916-923.

11 Martinez-Martin P, Schapira AH, Stocchi F, et al. Prevalence of nonmotor symptoms in Parkinson's disease in an international setting; study using nonmotor symptoms questionnaire in 545 patients. *Mov Disord* 2007;22:1623-1629.

12 Chaudhuri KR, Prieto-Jurcynska C, Naidu Y, et al. The nondeclaration of nonmotor symptoms of Parkinson's disease to health care professionals: an international study using the nonmotor symptoms questionnaire. *Mov Disord* 2010;25:697-701.

13 Wang G, Wan Y, Cheng Q, et al. Malnutrition and associated factors in Chinese patients with Parkinson's disease: Results from a pilot investigation. *Parkinsonism Relat Disord* 2010;16:119-123.

14 Cervantes-Arriaga A, Rodriguez-Violante M, Villar-Velarde A, Lopez-Gomez M, Corona T. [Metric properties of clinimetric indexes for non-motor dysfunction of Parkinson's disease in Mexican population.] *Rev Invest Clin* 2010;62:8-14.

15 Chaudhuri KR, Martinez-Martin P, Brown RG, et al. The metric properties of a novel non-motor symptoms scale for Parkinson's disease: Results from an international pilot study. *Mov Disord* 2007;22:1901-1911.

16 Honig H, Antonini A, Martinez-Martin P, et al. Intrajejunal levodopa infusion in Parkinson's disease: a pilot multicenter study of effects on nonmotor symptoms and quality of life. *Mov Disord* 2009;24:1468-1474.

17 Kim HJ, Park SY, Cho YJ, et al. Nonmotor symptoms in de novo Parkinson disease before and after dopaminergic treatment. *J Neurol Sci* 2009;287:200-204.

18 Martinez-Martin P, Rodriguez-Blazquez C, Abe K, et al. International study on the psychometric attributes of the non-motor symptoms scale in Parkinson disease. *Neurology* 2009;73:1584-1591.

19 Wang G, Hong Z, Cheng Q, et al. Validation of the Chinese Non-Motor Symptoms Scale for Parkinson's disease: Results from a Chinese pilot study. *Clin Neurol Neurosurgery* 2009;111:523-526.

20 Barone P, Antonini A, Colosimo C, et al. The PRIAMO study: A multicenter assessment of nonmotor symptoms and their impact on quality of life in Parkinson's disease. *Mov Disord* 2009;24:1641-1649.

21 Colosimo C, Morgante L, Antonini A, et al. Non-motor symptoms in atypical and secondary parkinsonism: the PRIAMO study. *J Neurol* 2010;257:5-14.

22 Hoehn MM, Yahr MD. Parkinsonism: onset, progression, and mortality. *Neurology* 1967;17:427-442.

23 Global Parkinson's Disease Survey Steering Committee. Factors impacting on quality of life in Parkinson's disease: results from an international survey. *Mov Disord* 2002;17:60-67.

24 Lohle M, Storch A, Reichmann H. Beyond tremor and rigidity: non-motor features of Parkinson's disease. *J Neural Transm* 2009;116:1483-1492.

25 Wolters EC. Non-motor extranigral signs and symptoms in Parkinson's disease. *Parkinsonism Relat Disord* 2009;15(suppl 3):S6-S12.

26 Qin Z, Zhang L, Sun F, et al. Health related quality of life in early Parkinson's disease: Impact of motor and non-motor symptoms, results from Chinese levodopa exposed cohort. *Parkinsonism. Rel Disord* 2009;15:767-771.

27 Chaudhuri KR, Healy, DG, Schapira AH. Non-motor symptoms of Parkinson's disease: diagnosis and management. *Lancet Neurol* 2006;5:235-245.

28 Miller E, Berrios GE, Politynska BE. Caring for someone with Parkinson's disease: factors that contribute to distress. *Int J Geriatr Psychiatry* 1998;11:263-268.

29 Carter JH, Stewart BJ, Archbold PG, et al. Living with a person who has Parkinson's disease: the spouse's perspective by stage of disease. *Mov Disord* 2004;13:20-28.

30 Meara J, Mitchelmore E, Hobson P. Use of the GDS-15 geriatric depression scale as a screening instrument for depressive symptomatology in patients with Parkinson's disease and their carers in the community. *Age Aging* 1999;28:35-38.

31 Habermann B. Spousal perspective of Parkinson's disease in middle life. *J Adv Nurs* 2000;31:1409-1415.

32 Fernandez HH, Tabamo REJ, David RR, Friedman JH. Predictors of depressive symptoms among spouse caregivers in Parkinson's disease. *Mov Disord* 2001;16:1123-1125.

33 Caap-Ahlgren M, Dehlin O. Factors of importance to the caregiver burden experienced by family caregivers of Parkinson's disease patients. *Aging Clin Exp Res* 2002;14:371-377.

34 Edwards NE, Scheetz PS. Predictors of burden for caregivers of patients with Parkinson's disease. *J Neurosci Nurs* 2002;34:184-190.

35 Happe S, Berger K. The association between caregiver burden and sleep disturbances in partners of patients with Parkinson's disease. *Age Ageing* 2002;31:349-354.

36 Thommessen B, Aarsland D, Braekhus A, Oksengaard AR, Engedal K, Laake K. The psychosocial burden on spouses of the elderly with stroke, dementia and Parkinson's disease. *Int J Geriatr Psychiatry* 2002;17:78-84.

37 Martinez-Martin P, Guerrero-Diaz MT, Frades-Payo B. [Neuropsychological disorders in Parkinson's disease: evaluating them and their impact on the caregiver]. *Rev Neurol* 2004;39:639-645.

38 Pal PK, Thennarasu K, Fleming J, Schulzer M, Brown T, Calne SM. Nocturnal sleep disturbances and daytime dysfunction in patients with Parkinson's disease and in their caregivers. *Parkinsonism Relat Disord* 2004;10:157-168.

39 Martinez-Martin P, Benito-Leon J, Alonso F, et al. Quality of life of caregivers in Parkinson's disease. *Qual Life Res* 2005;14:463-472.

40 Cifu DX, Carne W, Brown R, et al. Caregiver distress in parkinsonism. *J Rehabil Res Dev* 2006;43:499-508.

41 Schrag A, Hovris A, Morley D, Quinn N, Jahanshahi M. Caregiver-burden in Parkinson's disease is closely associated with psychiatric symptoms, falls, and disability. *Parkinsonism Relat Disord* 2006;12:35-41.

42 Schestatsky P, Zanatto VC, Margis R, et al. Quality of life in a Brazilian sample of patients with Parkinson's disease and their caregivers. *Rev Bras Psiquiatr* 2006;28:209-211.

43 Aarsland D, Bronnick K, Ehrt U, et al. Neuropsychiatric symptoms in patients with Parkinson's disease and dementia: frequency, profile and associated care giver stress. *J Neurol Neurosurg Psychiatry* 2007;78:36.

44 Kim KS, Kim BJ, Kim KH, et al. Subjective and objective caregiver burden in Parkinson's disease. *Taehan Kanho Hakhoe Chi* 2007;37:242-248.

45 Martinez-Martin P, Forjaz MJ, Frades-Payo B, et al. Caregiver burden in Parkinson's disease. *Mov Disord* 2007a;22:924-931.

46 Carter JH, Stewart BJ, Lyons, KS, Archbold, PG. Do motor and nonmotor symptoms in PD patients predict caregiver strain and depression? *Mov Disord* 2008;23:1211-1216.

47 Lokk J. Caregiver strain in Parkinson's disease and the impact of disease duration. Eur J Phys *Rehabil Med* 2008;44:39-45.

48 Martinez-Martin P, Arroyo S, Rojo-Abuin JM, Rodriguez-Blazquez C, Frades B, de Pedro CJ. Burden, perceived health status, and mood among caregivers of Parkinson's disease patients. *Mov Disord* 2008;23:1673-1680.

49 D'Amelio M, Terruso V, Palmeri B, et al. Predictors of caregiver burden in partners of patients with Parkinson's disease. *Neurol Sci* 2009;30:171-174.

50 Stella F, Banzato CE, Quagliato EM, Viana MA, Christofoletti G. Psychopathological features in patients with Parkinson's disease and related caregivers' burden. *Int J Geriatr Psychiatry* 2009;24:1158-1165.

51 Roland KP, Jenkins ME, Johnson AM. An exploration of the burden experienced by spousal caregivers of individuals with Parkinson's disease. *Mov Disord* 2010;25:189-193.

52 Ware JE Jr, Sherbourne CD. The MOS 36-item short-form health survey (SF-36): I. Conceptual framework and item selection. *Med Care* 1992;30:473-483.

53 EuroQol Group. EuroQol-a new facility for the measurement of health-related quality of life. *Health Policy* 1990;16:199-208.

54 WHOQOL Group. Development of the World Health Organization WHOQOL-BREF quality of life assessment. *Psychol Med* 1998;28:551-558.

55 Glozman JM, Bicheva KG, Fedorova NV. Scale of quality of life of care-givers (SQLC). *J Neurol* 1998;245:39-41.

56 Zarit SH, Reever KE, Bach-Peterson J. Relatives of the impaired elderly: correlates of feelings of burden. *Gerontologist* 1980;20:649-655.

57 Novak M, Guest C. Application of a multidimensional caregiver burden inventory. *The Gerontologist* 1989;29:798-803.

58 Montgomery RJV, Gonyea JG, Hooyman NR. Caregiving and the experience of subjective and objective burden. *Family Relations* 1985;34:19-26.

59 Olanow CW, Stern MB, Sethi K. The scientific and clinical basis for the treatment of Parkinson disease. *Neurology* 2009;72(suppl 4):1-136.

60 Goetz CG, Stebbins GT. Risk factors for nursing home placement in advanced Parkinson's disease. *Neurology* 1993;43:2227-2229.

61 Guttman M, Slaughter PM, Theriault ME, DeBoer DP, Naylor CD. Burden of parkinsonism: a population-based study. *Mov Disord* 2002;18:313-319.

62 Magerkurth C, Schnitzer R, Braune S. Symptoms of autonomic failure in Parkinson's disease: prevalence and impact on daily life. *Clin Autonom Res* 2005;15:76-82.

63 Findley L, Aujla M, Bain PG, et al. Direct economic impact of Parkinson's disease: a research survey in the United Kingdom. *Mov Disord* 2003;18:1139-1145.

64 Cubo E, Martinez-Martin P, Gonzalez M, Frades B, ELEP Group. Impact of motor and non-motor symptoms on the direct costs of Parkinson's disease [Spanish]. *Neurologia* 2009;24:15-23.

65 Dodel RC, Singer M, Kohne-Volland R, et al. The economic impact of Parkinson's disease: An estimation based on a 3-month prospective analysis. *Pharmacoeconomics* 1998;14:299-312.

66 Pålhagen S, Heinonen E, Hagglund J, Kaugesaar T, Maki-Ikola O, Palm R. Selegiline slows the progression of the symptoms of Parkinson disease. *Neurology* 2006;66:1200-1206.

67 Haycox A, Armand C, Murteira S, Cochran J, François C. Cost effectiveness of rasagiline and pramipexole as treatment strategies in early Parkinson's disease in the UK setting: An economic Markov model evaluation. *Drugs Aging* 2009;26:791-801.

68 Parkinson Study Group. A controlled, randomized, delayed-start study of rasagiline in early Parkinson disease. *Arch Neurol* 2004;61:561-566.

69 Olanow CW, Rascol O, Hauser R, et al. A double-blind, delayed-start trial of rasagiline in Parkinson's disease. *N Engl J Med* 2009a;361:1268-1278.

70 Poewe W, Hauser R, Lang AE. Rasagiline 1 mg/day provides benefits in the progression of non-motor symptoms in patients with early Parkinson's disease: Assessment with the revised MDS-UPDRS. *Mov Disord* 2009;24:S272-S273.

Chapter 3

Assessing non-motor symptoms: an overview of scales and questionnaires

Carmen Rodriguez-Blazquez, Madhuja Tanya Mitra and
Pablo Martinez-Martin

Introduction

The NMSs of Parkinson's disease (PD) have been an under-recognized part of PD, often leading to a poor quality of life for patients and their caregivers [1]. NMSs are common, with incidence and severity varying widely from patient to patient. It has been found that their incidence significantly increases with disease severity – monitored using Hoehn and Yahr (H&Y) staging [2]. Studies have shown that NMSs such as depression or constipation may precede the motor signs of PD [3,4]. Therefore, this relatively newly recognized but significant aspect of PD requires NMS declaration by patients and evaluation by health care professionals in order to determine its presence and monitor its severity. Assessment of NMSs can be performed through a variety of scales and questionnaires which this chapter will focus on.

The importance of assessing non-motor symptoms

NMS assessment is essential to monitor progression and/or potential response to treatment as well as the effect on patient's HRQoL [5]. Despite the importance of recognizing NMSs in PD, studies have shown

K. R. Chaudhuri et al., *Handbook of Non-Motor Symptoms
in Parkinson's Disease*, DOI: 10.1007/978-1-908517-60-9_3,
© Springer Healthcare, a part of Springer Science+Business Media 2011

that neurologists fail to identify them in over 50% of consultations [6]. An international study [1] discovered that patients often fail to disclose NMSs, with delusions, daytime sleepiness, intense and vivid dreams, and dizziness being the most non-declared symptoms.

Under-recognition and non-disclosure of NMSs can act as barriers to treatment. These can be overcome by routinely using assessment scales in the clinical setting. Treatment is available for most NMSs and can greatly improve patient-related quality of life HRQoL, so assessment and awareness of NMSs are vital to improve patient care [1].

General scales for assessment of non-motor symptoms in Parkinson's disease

A wide variety of scales have been used to assess NMSs in PD (the most important of them are listed in Figure 3.1) [24]. However, some of these were not specifically designed for use in PD patients and they lack adaptation and validation in this population. Recently, a set of specific NMS measures, which are reviewed here, have been developed.

The Movement Disorder Society Unified Parkinson's Disease Rating Scale

The Unified Parkinson's Disease Rating Scale (UPDRS) is one of the most widely used scales measuring motor symptoms in PD patients [25]. Although the scale had good clinical application and comprehensive coverage, it included very few screening questions on non-motor elements of PD [25]. The Movement Disorder Society (MDS) sponsored a revision of the UPDRS, called the MDS-UPDRS [26,27], which included modifications that integrated the non-motor aspects of the disease with NMSs such as anxiety, urinary problems, constipation, fatigue and sleep disturbances [26]. The MDS-UPDRS [27] is structured as follows:

I. Non-motor Experiences of Daily Living
II. Motor Experiences of Daily Living
III. Motor Examination
IV. Motor Complications.

Several questions in Part I and all of Part II are completed by the patient and/or caregiver. The total time to complete the MDS-UPDRS should be approximately 30 minutes [26]. In a first validation study, it was found to have good combined clinimetric results that support the reliability and validity of the scale [27].

The SCOPA set (cognition, autonomic, sleep and psychiatric complications)

The SCales for Outcomes in PArkinson's Disease – Cognition (SCOPA-COG) was developed as a tool for assessing cognitive deficits specific to PD [28]. The scale consists of 10 items with a maximum score of 43, with higher scores reflecting better performance [28]. The SCOPA-COG demonstrated good consistency, reliability and validity [28]. In addition, it has been shown to better detect individual cognitive differences than other scales (specifically the MMSE and CAMCOG) [28], and takes only

Some instruments applied to assess non-motor symptoms in Parkinson's disease	
NMS domain	**Instruments**
Cognitive impairment	Mini-Mental State Examination (MMSE) [7]
	Mattis Dementia Rating Scale (DRS) [8]
Depression	Hamilton Depression Scale (Ham-D) [9]
	Beck Depression Inventory (BDI) [10]
	Hospital Anxiety and Depression Scale (HADS) [11]
Anxiety	Hamilton Anxiety Rating Scale (HARS) [12]
	Zung Self-rating Anxiety Scale (SAS) [13]
	Hospital Anxiety and Depression Scale (HADS) [11]
Apathy	Apathy Scale (AS) [14]
	Lille Apathy Rating Scale (LARS) [15]
Anhedonia	Snaith–Hamilton Pleasure Scale (SHAPS) [16]
Psychotic symptoms	Parkinson Psychiatric Rating Scale (PPRS) [17]
Sleep disorder	Pittsburgh Sleep Quality Index (PSQI) [18]
	Epworth Sleepiness Scale (ESS) [19]
	Parkinson's Disease Sleep Scale (PDSS) [20]
Fatigue	Fatigue Impact Scale for Daily Use (D-FIS) [21]
	Parkinson Fatigue Scale (PFS-16) [22]
Pain	McGill Pain Questionnaire [23]

Figure 3.1 Some instruments applied to assess non-motor symptoms in Parkinson's disease. NMS, non-motor symptoms. Adapted from Martinez-Martin et al 2009 [24].

10–15 minutes to complete [29]. The limitations of this scale include that it assesses only 'frontal–subcortical' functioning [29]. Large prospective studies found that the SCOPA-COG was affected by patient age, education level, age at disease onset and duration of disease [30–32].

Dysautonomia symptoms (eg, orthostatism, constipation, excessive sweating, bladder dysfunction) have been commonly described in PD patients [33]. These symptoms are physically as well as socially disabling for patients and can exacerbate other NMS problems such as sleep disturbance [34]. The SCOPA – Autonomic (SCOPA-AUT) is a specific scale designed to assess autonomic dysfunction in PD patients [35]. It is valid, sensitive and reliable [36], and thus is one of the two scales that meet the 'recommended' criteria for dysautonomia assessment by the MDS (the other is the NMSQuest) [33]. However, improvements to the scale would allow measurement of more subtle dysautonomic symptoms and make it shorter [37].

Sleep disorders in PD are a common problem for patients, with community-based studies reporting prevalence in up to 60% of PD patients [38]. Disturbances include restless legs, insomnia, excessive daytime sleepiness and rapid eye movement (REM) sleep behavior disorder (RBD) [39]. The SCOPA-Sleep (SCOPA-S) is a disease-specific rating scale for assessing these disorders [40]. It has been reported to provide valid, reliable, and useful means to evaluate sleep disorders in PD [40,41]. SCOPA-S assesses nocturnal sleep disorders and daytime somnolence, detecting differences between individuals better than the Pittsburgh Sleep Quality Index and the Epworth Sleepiness Scale [40]. However, it does not explore the potential causes of the problems [41].

Psychotic symptom assessment is the objective of the SCOPA – Psychiatric Complications (SCOPA-PC) [42]. The SCOPA-PC is a version of the Parkinson Psychiatric Rating Scale (PPRS) [17], with changes in the response options and an item on compulsive behavior in PD. It is composed of seven items on hallucinations, illusions, paranoid ideation, altered dream phenomena, confusion, sexual preoccupation and compulsive behavior, which are scored on a scale from 0 (no symptoms) to 3 (severe symptoms). It has been found to be reliable, valid and is easily administered [42].

Use of quality of-life scales for the assessment of non-motor symptoms

Some of the most frequently used QoL scales in PD include questions specifically addressed to measure the impact of NMSs, because they have been identified as the main predictors of poor QoL in PD patients [43]. This is the case of the Parkinson's Disease Questionnaire – 39 items (PDQ-39) [44,45] and the Parkinson's Disease Quality of Life (PDQL) questionnaire [46].

The Parkinson's Disease Questionnaire – 39 items

The PDQ-39 is a self-administered measure of subjective health status [44,45]. The 39 items of which it is composed are grouped in eight sub-scales: mobility, activities of daily living (ADL), emotional wellbeing, stigma, social support, cognition, communication and bodily discomfort. Responses are scored in a scale from 0 (never) to 4 (always). A summary index (SI) is calculated as the mean of the domain scores, with higher scores meaning a lower QoL.

Grosset et al [47] suggest that PDQ-39 performs as an indirect indicator of NMSs in PD. In fact, PDQ-39 correlates strongly with a global measure of NMSs such as the NMSS [48]. It also correlates with scales measuring specific NMSs, including depression [49,50], dysautonomia [51] and fatigue [52].

The PDQ-39 can also estimate the impact of NMSs in PD patients [43]. Finally, some NMSs such as depression, fatigue, urinary incontinence, headache and pain have been found to be predictors of PDQ-39 scores [49,53,54].

The Parkinson's Disease Quality of Life Questionnaire

The PDQL [46] is composed of 37 items, grouped in 4 subscales:
- parkinsonian symptoms (14 items),
- systemic symptoms (7 items),
- social function (7 items), and
- emotional function (9 items).

Answer options range from 1 (all of the time) to 5 (never), and PDQL SI ranges from 37 to 185, with higher scores reflecting better QoL.

The PDQL has proved to be an acceptable, reliable, valid and precise instrument for use in PD [50]. It can also predict health-care use [55] and is responsive to changes in PD – due to either treatment or disease progression [56–59]. Although more than half the items are related to NMSs, the PDQL does not cover in depth several areas such as mental health, social function and sleep.

Non-motor symptom-specific scales

In recent years, two instruments have been designed and validated to measure NMSs in PD patients in a global, comprehensive way: the Non-Motor Symptoms Questionnaire (NMSQuest) [60] and the Non-Motor Symptoms Scale (NMSS) [5,50].

The NMSQuest is a 30-item self-completed screening tool, with a 'yes/no' response format. It was designed to draw attention to the presence of NMSs, empowering patients to disclose non-motor manifestations otherwise unrecognized [1], and to prompt health professionals to initiate further investigation and intervention. The items were derived from the previous literature, expert consultation, and nurse and patient group opinions. The NMSQuest asks about the presence of NMSs over the last month, and the average time taken to complete it is 5–7 minutes. It has proved its usefulness for NMS screening [2,60]. The NMSQuest showed a significant association with H&Y stage and age, with total number of NMSs increasing in patients in more advanced stages and in older patients [2]. The sleep-related items of the NMSQuest correlated with the Parkinson's Disease Sleep Scale (PDSS) and sleep log scores [61]. Finally, the NMSQuest has been recommended by the Movement Disorders Task Force on dysautonomia rating scales for Parkinson's disease [33].

The NMSS is reviewed in depth in Chapter 4.

References

1   Chaudhuri KR, Prieto-Jurcynska C, Naidu Y, et al. The nondeclaration of nonmotor symptoms of Parkinson's disease to health care professionals: an international study using the nonmotor symptoms questionnaire. *Mov Disord* 2010;25:697-701.
2   Martinez-Martin P, Schapira AH, Stocchi F, et al. Prevalence of nonmotor symptoms in Parkinson's disease in an international setting; study using nonmotor symptoms questionnaire in 545 patients. *Mov Disord* 2007;22:1623-1629.

3   Braak H, Del Tredici K, Rub U, de Vos RA, Jansen Steur EN, Braak E. Staging of brain pathology related to sporadic Parkinson's disease. *Neurobiol Aging* 2003;24:197-211.

4   Chaudhuri KR, Healy DG, Schapira AH. Non-motor symptoms of Parkinson's disease: diagnosis and management. *Lancet Neurol* 2006;5:235-245.

5   Chaudhuri KR, Martinez-Martin P, Brown RG, et al. The metric properties of a novel non-motor symptoms scale for Parkinson's disease: Results from an international pilot study. *Mov Disord* 2007;22:1901-1911.

6   Shulman LM, Taback RL, Rabinstein AA, Weiner WJ. Non-recognition of depression and other non-motor symptoms in Parkinson's disease. *Parkinsonism Relat Disord* 2002;8:193-197.

7   Folstein MF, Folstein SE, McHugh PR. Mini-mental state. A practical method for grading the cognitive state of patients for the clinician. *J Psychiatr Res* 1975;12:189-198.

8   Mattis S. Mental status examination for organic mental syndrome in the elderly patient. In: Bellak L, Karasu TB (eds), *Geriatric Psychiatry: A Handbook for Psychiatrists and Primary Care Physicians*. New York: Grune & Stratton, 1976: 77-121.

9   Hamilton M. A rating scale for depression. *J Neurol Neurosurg Psychiatry* 1960;23:56-62.

10   Beck AT, Ward CH, Mendelson M, Mock J, Erbaugh J. An inventory for measuring depression. *Arch Gen Psychiatry* 1961;4:561-571.

11   Zigmond AS, Snaith RP. The Hospital Anxiety and Depression Scale. *Acta Psychiatr Scand* 1983;67:361-370.

12   Hamilton M. The assessment of anxiety states by rating. Br J Med Psychol 1959;32:50-55.

13   Zung WWK. A rating instrument for anxiety disorders. *Psychosomatics* 1971;12:371-379.

14   Starkstein SE, Mayberg HS, Preziosi TJ, Andrezejewski P, Leiguarda R, Robinson RG. Reliability, validity, and clinical correlates of apathy in Parkinson's disease. *J Neuropsychiatry Clin Neurosci* 1992;4:134-139.

15   Sockeel P, Dujardin K, Devos D, Deneve C, Destee A, Defebvre L. The Lille apathy rating scale (LARS). a new instrument for detecting and quantifying apathy: validation in Parkinson's disease. *J Neurol Neurosurg Psychiatry* 2006;77:579-584.

16   Snaith RP, Hamilton M, Morley S, Humayan A, Hargreaves D, Trigwell P. A scale for the assessment of hedonic tone: the Snaith-Hamilton Pleasure Scale. *Br J Psychiatry* 1995;167:99-103.

17   Friedberg G, Zoldan J, Weizman A, Melamed E. Parkinson Psychosis Rating Scale: a practical instrument for grading psychosis in Parkinson's disease. *Clin Neuropharmacol* 1998;21:280-284.

18   Buysse DJ, Reynolds III CF, Monk TH, Berman SR, Kupfer DJ. The Pittsburgh Sleep Quality Index: a new instrument for psychiatric practice and research. *Psychiatry Res* 1989;28:193-213.

19   Johns MW. A new method for measuring daytime sleepiness: the Epworth sleepiness scale. *Sleep* 1991;14:540-545.

20   Chaudhuri KR, Pal S, DiMarco A, et al. The Parkinson's disease sleep scale: a new instrument for assessing sleep and nocturnal disability in Parkinson's disease. *J Neurol Neurosurg Psychiatry* 2002;73:629-635.

21   Fisk JD, Doble SE. Construction and validation of a fatigue impact scale for daily administration (D-FIS). *Qual Life Res* 2002;11:263-272.

22   Brown RG, Dittner A, Findley L, Wessely SC. The Parkinson fatigue scale. *Parkinsonism Relat Disord* 2005;11:49-55.

23   Lee MA, Walker RW, Hildreth TJ, Prentice WM. A survey of pain in idiopathic Parkinson's disease. *J Pain Symptom Manag* 2006;32:462-469.

24   Martinez-Martin P, Marinus J, van Hilten B. Assessment tools for non-motor symptoms of Parkinson's Disease. In: Chaudhuri KR, Tolosa E, Schapira A, Poewe W (eds), *Non-Motor Symptoms of Parkinson's Disease*. Oxford: Oxford University Press, 2009: 47-58.

25   Movement Disorders Society Task Force. The Unified Parkinson's Disease Rating Scale (UPDRS): status and recommendations. *Mov Disord* 2003;18:738-750.

26   Goetz CG, Fahn S, Martinez-Martin P, et al. Movement Disorder Society-sponsored revision of the Unified Parkinson's Disease Rating Scale (MDS-UPDRS): Process, format, and clinimetric testing plan. *Mov Disord* 2007;22:41-47.

27 Goetz CG, Tilley BC, Shaftman SR, et al. Movement Disorder Society-sponsored revision of the Unified Parkinson's Disease Rating Scale (MDS-UPDRS): scale presentation and clinimetric testing results. *Mov Disord* 2008;23:2129-2170.

28 Marinus J, Visser M, Verwey NA, et al. Assessment of cognition in Parkinson's disease. *Neurology* 2003;61:1222-1228.

29 Kulisevsky J, Pagonabarraga J. Cognitive impairment in Parkinson's disease: tools for diagnosis and assessment. *Mov Disord* 2009;24:1103-1110.

30 Verbaan D, Marinus J, Visser M, et al. Cognitive impairment in Parkinson's disease. *J Neurol Neurosurg Psychiatry* 2007;78:1182-1187.

31 Carod-Artal FJ, Martinez-Martin P, Kummer W, Ribeiro LS. Psychometric attributes of the SCOPACOG Brazilian version. *Mov Disord* 2008;23:81-87.

32 Martinez-Martin P, Frades-Payo B, Rodriguez-Blazquez C, Forjaz MJ, Pedro-Cuesta J, Grupo Estudio Longitudinal de Pacientes con Enfermedad de Parkinson. [Psychometric attributes of Scales for Outcomes in Parkinson's Disease - Cognition (SCOPA-Cog). Castilian language]. *Rev Neurol* 2008;47:337-343.

33 Evatt ML, Chaudhuri KR, Chou KL, et al. Dysautonomia rating scales in Parkinson's disease: sialorrhea, dysphagia, and constipation - critique and recommendations by movement disorders task force on rating scales for Parkinson's disease. *Mov Disord* 2009;24:635-646.

34 Mitra T, Chaudhuri KR. Sleep dysfunction and role of dysautonomia in Parkinson's disease. *Parkinsonism Relat Disord* 2009;15(suppl 3):S93-S95.

35 Visser M, Marinus J, Stiggelbout AM, van Hilten JJ. Assessment of autonomic dysfunction in Parkinson's disease: the SCOPA-AUT. *Mov Disord* 2004;19:1306-1312.

36 Rodriguez-Blazquez C, Forjaz MJ, Frades-Payo B, Pedro-Cuesta J, Martinez-Martin P. Independent validation of the scales for outcomes in Parkinson's disease - autonomic (SCOPA-AUT). *Eur J Neurol* 2010;17:194-201.

37 Forjaz MJ, Ayala A, Rodriguez-Blazquez C, Frades-Payo B, Martinez-Martin P. Assessing autonomic symptoms of Parkinson's disease with the SCOPA-AUT: a new perspective from Rasch analysis. *Eur J Neurol* 2010;17:273-279.

38 Tandberg E, Larsen JP, Karlsen K. Excessive daytime sleepiness and sleep benefit in Parkinson's disease: a community-based study. *Mov Disord* 1999;14:922-927.

39 Menza M, Dobkin RD, Marin H, Bienfait K. Sleep disturbances in Parkinson's disease. *Mov Disord* 2010;25(suppl 1):S117-S122.

40 Marinus J, Visser M, van Hilten JJ, Lammers GJ, Stiggelbout AM. Assessment of sleep and sleepiness in Parkinson disease. *Sleep* 2003;26:1049-1054.

41 Martinez-Martin P, Visser M, Rodriguez-Blazquez C, Marinus J, Chaudhuri KR, van Hilten JJ. SCOPAsleep and PDSS: two scales for assessment of sleep disorder in Parkinson's disease. *Mov Disord* 2008;23:1681-1688.

42 Visser M, Verbaan D, van Rooden SM, Stiggelbout AM, Marinus J, van Hilten JJ. Assessment of psychiatric complications in Parkinson's disease: The SCOPA-PC. *Mov Disord* 2007;22:2221-2228.

43 Barone P, Antonini A, Colosimo C, et al. The PRIAMO study: A multicenter assessment of nonmotor symptoms and their impact on quality of life in Parkinson's disease. *Mov Disord* 2009;24:1641-1649.

44 Jenkinson C, Peto V, Fitzpatrick R, Greenhall R, Hyman N. Self-reported functioning and well-being in patients with Parkinson's disease: Comparison of the Short-form Health Survey (SF-36) and the Parkinson's Disease Questionnaire (PDQ-39). *Age Aging* 1995;24:505-509.

45 Peto V, Jenkinson C, Fitzpatrick R, Greenhall R. The development and validation of a short measure of functioning and well being for individuals with Parkinson's disease. *Qual Life Res* 1995;4:241-248.

46 de Boer AG, Wijker W, Speelman JD, de Haes JC. Quality of life in patients with Parkinson's disease: development of a questionnaire. *J Neurol Neurosurg Psychiatry* 1996;61:70-74.

47 Grosset D, Taurah L, Burn DJ, et al. A multicentre longitudinal observational study of changes in self reported health status in people with Parkinson's disease left untreated at diagnosis. *J Neurol Neurosurg Psychiatry* 2007;78:465-469.

48 Martinez-Martin P, Serrano-Duenas M, Forjaz MJ, Serrano MS. Two questionnaires for Parkinson's disease: are the PDQ-39 and PDQL equivalent? *Qual Life Res* 2007;16:1221-1230.

49 Schrag A, Jahanshahi M, Quinn N. What contributes to quality of life in patients with Parkinson's disease? *J Neurol Neurosurg Psychiatry* 2000;69:308-312.

50 Martinez-Martin P, Rodriguez-Blazquez C, Abe K, et al. International study on the psychometric attributes of the non-motor symptoms scale in Parkinson disease. *Neurology* 2009;73:1584-1591.

51 Carod-Artal FJ, da Silveira RL, Kummer W, Martinez-Martin P. Psychometric properties of the SCOPA-AUT Brazilian Portuguese version. *Mov Disord* 2010;25:205-212.

52 Herlofson K, Larsen JP. The influence of fatigue on health-related quality of life in patients with Parkinson's disease. *Acta Neurol Scand* 2003;107:1-6.

53 Global Parkinson's Disease Survey Steering Committee. Factors impacting on quality of life in Parkinson's disease: results from an international survey. *Mov Disord* 2002;17:60-67.

54 Rahman S, Griffin HJ, Quinn NP, Jahanshahi M. Quality of life in Parkinson's disease: the relative importance of the symptoms. *Mov Disord* 2008;23:1428-1434.

55 de Boer AG, Sprangers MA, Speelman HD, de Haes HC. Predictors of health care use in patients with Parkinson's disease: a longitudinal study. *Mov Disord* 1999;14:772-779.

56 Fraix V, Houeto JL, Lagrange C, et al. Clinical and economic results of bilateral subthalamic nucleus stimulation in Parkinson's disease. *J Neurol Neurosurg Psychiatry* 2006;77:443-449.

57 Reuther M, Spottke EA, Klotsche J, et al. Assessing health-related quality of life in patients with Parkinson's disease in a prospective longitudinal study. *Parkinsonism Relat Disord* 2007;13:108-114.

58 Schrag A, Spottke A, Quinn NP, Dodel R. Comparative responsiveness of Parkinson's disease scales to change over time. *Mov Disord* 2009;24:813-818.

59 Yousefi B, Tadibi V, Khoei AF, Montazeri A. Exercise therapy, quality of life, and activities of daily living in patients with Parkinson disease: a small scale quasi-randomised trial. *Trials* 2009;10:67.

60 Chaudhuri KR, Martinez-Martin P, Schapira AH, et al. International multicenter pilot study of the first comprehensive self-completed nonmotor symptoms questionnaire for Parkinson's disease: the NMSQuest study. *Mov Disord* 2006;21:916-923.

61 Perez-Lloret S, Rossi M, Cardinali DP, Merello M. Validation of the sleep related items of the Nonmotor Symptoms Questionnaire for Parkinson's disease (NMSQuest). *Parkinsonism Relat Disord* 2008;14:641-645.

Chapter 4

An in-depth look at the Non-Motor Symptom Scale

Monica Kurtis, Kartik Logishetty and Pablo Martinez-Martin

Aims of the scale

To provide a fast and reliable tool to measure the whole burden of non-motor symptoms in Parkinson's disease

The Non-Motor Symptoms Scale (NMSS) was developed in 2006 to provide clinicians with an instrument for assessment of non-motor symptoms (NMSs) in patients with Parkinson's disease (PD) [1]. This validated instrument categorizes NMSs into 30 questions in nine domains. The scale estimates the impact of NMSs by weighing each symptom by frequency and severity, thus capturing their global burden for patients.

The NMSS provides a complementary tool after screening for NMSs with the Non-Motor Symptom Questionnaire (NMSQuest). This scale is the first comprehensive, holistic and practical measuring tool to ascertain the wide range of NMS symptoms in PD. It provides a quantitative measure that captures infrequent but severe symptoms such as hallucinations and less serious but frequent symptoms such as fatigue and constipation.

To bring attention to non-motor symptoms in Parkinson's disease

The range of NMSs seen in PD has historically been neglected by both clinicians and patients. During their check-ups, patients often do not report pain, sleep problems, constipation or other NMSs spontane-

K. R. Chaudhuri et al., *Handbook of Non-Motor Symptoms in Parkinson's Disease*, DOI: 10.1007/978-1-908517-60-9_4, © Springer Healthcare, a part of Springer Science+Business Media 2011

ously. This may be because they do not relate these symptoms to their PD or may be too embarrassed to discuss them. The non-declaration of NMSs to health-care professionals was recently highlighted in a study including 242 PD patients (Hoehn and Yahr [H&Y] 1–5, ages 34–91 years). Investigators found that the mean number of undeclared NMSs was 4.6 [2].

Instead, clinicians tend to concentrate their time and effort on the more apparent motor symptoms, thus underdiagnosing NMSs. In a prospective study in patients with PD, neurologists failed to diagnose depression, anxiety, fatigue and sleep disturbance in 40–75% of patients during routine office visits [3]. Furthermore, neurologists may not educate and inform patients about potential NMSs at diagnosis and follow-up. One of the aims of the NMSS is to create a platform for dialogue between the patient and health-care provider about NMSs in PD, so that they may be reported, recognized and addressed.

To provide a holistic assessment of the Parkinson's disease patient

The NMSS is complementary to the motor evaluation of PD patients. In the future, it may be proposed as an annex to the new MDS-UPDRS (Movement Disorders Society Unified Parkinson's Disease Rating Scale). It has only recently been recognized that the burden of NMSs significantly affects patients' perception of well-being. Multiple studies have stressed the importance of depression, fatigue, daytime sleepiness and dysautonomia as factors that predict patients' health-related quality of life (HRQoL) [4–10]. Recent data have demonstrated that the NMSS total score has a higher correlation with HRQoL than motor scores [11]. Therefore, it should be compulsory that the PD patient be quantitatively assessed for NMSs at the initial evaluation and at follow-up.

To plan effective treatment

One of the most pressing challenges in PD today is the development of effective treatments for NMSs. This scale's sensitivity allows the clinician to quantify treatment effects by calculating relative change and effect size.

History of the development and validation of the Non-Motor Symptoms Scale

Recognizing a void and a need

Instruments to assess individual NMSs, such as sleep, depression, and autonomic and cognitive functions, have existed for some time in clinical neurology. However, until recently, there was no single instrument that could provide a holistic assessment of the range of NMSs in PD. In 2004, an international, multidisciplinary group of experts (including clinicians, researchers, nurses and patient-group representatives) collaborated to develop a comprehensive instrument to evaluate the wide range of NMSs in PD. The challenges were many: it had to be practical, reliable, valid, sensitive to change and interpretable in different languages. This first meeting of the Parkinson's Disease Non Motor Group (PD-NMG) planted the seed for the development of the following [12]:

- the Non-Motor Symptom Assessment Questionnaire (NMQuest)
- the Non-Motor Symptom Scale (NMSS).

Drafting the NMSS

The NMSS was initially divided into 10 major domains containing 32 questions, based on a detailed literature review, expert experience, a patient response survey and evaluation of NMSQuest data, which led to the incorporation of four new items (diplopia, sweating, weight change and taste/smell) [12]. The scale aimed to be practical and quantitative, encompassing the whole range of NMSs experienced by people with PD. It envisaged that health-care professionals would administer the scale. Patients' responses would enable quantification of symptoms based on a multiple of severity (from 0 to 3) and frequency scores (from 1 to 4). Thus, the scale would pick up symptoms that were severe but infrequent, such as hallucinations, or not severe but persistent, such as fatigue, apathy and constipation [13].

The final version of NMSS is divided into 30 questions grouped in nine domains:

1. Cardiovascular: 2 items
2. Sleep/fatigue: 4 items
3. Mood/apathy: 6 items

4. Perceptual problems: 3 items
5. Attention/memory: 3 items
6. Gastrointestinal: 3 items
7. Urinary: 3 items
8. Sexual function: 2 items
9. Miscellaneous: 4 items.

Item questions are scored as a multiple of severity and frequency and domains are individually weighed.

Validating the NMSS

The first pilot study of clinimetric validation of the NMSS involved 242 PD outpatients across all age groups [1]. The sleep domain had the highest score, followed by mood/apathy and urinary system dominions. Most patients scored >50 on the scale, with an average of 56, range 0–243. Looking at the scale's convergent validity (ie, its ability to correlate with other measures), a very high correlation was found with quality of life and the NMSQuest. These findings suggest that the questionnaire correctly predicts NMSs, which are then picked up quantitatively by the scale. Assessments of the NMSS show that most domains, despite the complexity of the construct, have reasonable clinimetric properties, including stability [14].

Based on international collaboration, a second study testing the psychometric attributes of the NMSS scale on 411 PD patients was published recently. For domains, the Cronbach α-coefficient ranged from 0.44 to 0.85. The intraclass correlation coefficient (0.90 for the total score, 0.67–0.91 for domains) and Lin concordance coefficient (0.88) suggested satisfactory reproducibility. The NMSS total score correlated significantly with the SCales for Outcomes in PArkinson's disease (SCOPA) – Autonomic, Parkison's Disease Questionnaire (PDQ)-39 and EQ-5D (Spearman $r = 0.57$–0.70). Association was close between NMSS domains and the corresponding SCOPA – Autonomic domains ($r_s = 0.51$–0.65) and also with scales measuring related constructs (Parkinson's Disease Sleep Scale [PDSS], SCOPA-PC) (all $p < 0.0001$). The standard error of measurement was 13.91 for total score, ranging between 1.71 and 4.73 for domains [15]. The results of this muticenter, international effort demonstrated that the NMSS is an acceptable, reproducible, valid and precise assessment instrument for NMSs in PD, devoid of floor or ceiling effects.

Validated translations of the NMSS exist for Chinese- and German-speaking populations [16,17] and other language versions will be available in the near future.

Using the Non-Motor Symptom Scale in clinical practice and research

Monitoring treatment of the non-motor symptoms

There is a significant association between an increased NMSS score and disease progression, increased burden of NMSs and decreased health-related quality of life [18]. This robust correlation is seen in both treated and drug-naïve patients [19]. In clinical practice, the NMSS is thus a valid assessment tool for detecting NMSs and measuring treatment efficacy [14,15,20], particularly when used in tandem with the NMSQuest. The NMSS has also been suggested for the assessment of dysautonomia in PD [21].

To date, the NMSS has been used to demonstrate treatment efficacy in a few studies. A study by Simkin and colleagues [22] indicated that subthalamic nucleus deep brain stimulation in PD produces a reduction in NMS burden. Data from Kim and colleagues [23] confirmed the prevalence of NMSs in untreated new PD patients, and suggested that dopaminergic medication does not ameliorate these symptoms. This contrasts with Honig and colleagues' findings [20], which showed that intrajejunal levodopa infusion in patients with advanced PD improved NMSs and HRQoL at 6 months.

The effect of dopaminergic therapy on NMSs in PD remains questionable. Future intervention studies should apply the NMSS to clarify how currently available and future anti-parkinsonian treatments affect NMSs. It is possible that some NMS domains improve with treatment, but it is also well known that some secondary drug effects may aggravate symptoms such as hallucinations and sleepiness.

Biomarker in preclinical states

The NMSS may also be useful as a screening tool to detect PD biomarkers present in the preclinical/premotor state. It has been proposed that Lewy bodies in the lower brain stem and olfactory bulb initiate the pathological process of PD, with degeneration of dopaminergic neurons in the substantia nigra occurring much later [24]. This is reflected in NMSs including preclinical olfactory changes, sleep disturbances, constipation, and anxiety and depression, several years before the onset of motor symptoms [25]. Recent large trials have suggested that pharmacological therapies for PD, including pramipexole, ropinirole and rasagiline, may be neuroprotective or disease modifying [26–29], although the findings remain controversial [30]. In the near future, the NMSS may help establish a premotor diagnosis and thus provide an ideal population for clinical trials with drugs aimed at slowing disease progression.

Research of non-motor symptom pathways
Finally, the NMSS may provide fresh insight into the pathophysiology of the different NMSs found in PD and other parkinsonisms. It provides a quantifiable objective measuring tool that can be correlated with neurophysiology studies, as well as with anatomical and functional neuroimaging findings.

References

1   Chaudhuri KR, Martinez-Martin P, Brown RG, et al. The metric properties of a novel non-motor symptoms scale for Parkinson's disease: Results from an international pilot study. *Mov Disord* 2007;22:1901-1911.
2   Chaudhuri KR, Prieto-Jurcynska C, Naidu Y, et al. The Nondeclaration of Nonmotor Symptoms of Parkinson's Disease to Health Care Professionals: An International Study Using the Nonmotor Symptoms Questionnaire. *Mov Disord* 2010;25:704-709.
3   Shulman LM, Taback RL, Rabinstein AA, Weiner WJ. Non-recognition of depression and other nonmotor symptoms in Parkinson's disease. *Parkinsonism Relat Disord* 2002;8:193-197.
4   Schrag A, Jahanshahi M, Quinn N. What contributes to quality of life in patients with Parkinson's disease? *J Neurol Neurosurg Psychiatry* 2000;69:308-312.
5   Herlofson K, Larsen JP. The influence of fatigue on health-related quality of life in patients with Parkinson's disease. *Acta Neurol Scand* 2003;107:1-6.
6   Martinez-Martin P, Catalan MJ, Benito-Leon J, et al. Impact of fatigue in Parkinson's disease: the Fatigue Impact Scale for Daily Use (D-FIS). *Qual Life Res* 2006;15:597-606.
7   Marras C, McDermott MP, Rochon PA, Tanner CM, Naglie G, Lang AE. Predictors of deterioration in health-related quality of life in Parkinson's disease: results from the DATATOP trial. *Mov Disord* 2008;23:653-659.
8   Rahman S, Griffin HJ, Quinn NP, Jahanshahi M. Quality of life in Parkinson's disease: the relative importance of the symptoms. *Mov Disord* 2008;23:1428-1434.
9   Barone P, Antonini A, Colosimo C, et al. The PRIAMO study: A multicenter assessment of nonmotor symptoms and their impact on quality of life in Parkinson's disease. *Mov Disord* 2009;24:1641-1649.

10 Qin Z, Zhang L, Sun F, et al. Health related quality of life in early Parkinson's disease: impact of motor and non-motor symptoms, results from Chinese levodopa exposed cohort. *Parkinsonism Relat Disord* 2009;15:767-771.

11 Martinez-Martin P, Rodriguez-Blazquez C, Kurtis MM, et al. The Impact of Non Motor Symptoms on Health-Related Quality of Life of Patients with Parkinson's Disease. *Mov Disord* 2011; 26:399-406.

12 Chaudhuri KR, Schapira AHV, Martinez-Martin P, et al. Can we improve the holistic assessment of Parkinson's disease? The development of a non-motor symptom questionnaire and scale for Parkinson's disease. *Adv Clin Neurosci Rehabil* 2004;4:20-25.

13 Chaudhuri KR, Yates L, Martinez-Martin P. The non-motor symptom complex of parkinson's disease: a comprehensive assessment is essential. *Curr Neurol Neurosci Rep* 2005;5:275.

14 Chaudhuri KR, Martinez-Martin P. Quantitation of non-motor symptoms in Parkinson's disease. *Eur J Neurol* 2008;15(suppl 2):2-7.

15 Martinez-Martin P, Rodriguez-Blazquez C, Abe K, et al. International study on the psychometric attributes of the Non-Motor Symptoms Scale in Parkinson disease. *Neurology* 2009;73:1584-1591.

16 Wang G, Hong Z, Cheng Q, et al. Validation of the Chinese non-motor symptoms scale for Parkinson's disease: results from a Chinese pilot study. *Clin Neurol Neurosurg* 2009;111:523-526.

17 Storch A, Odin P, Trender-Gerhard I, et al. Non-motor Symptoms Questionnaire and Scale for Parkinson's disease: Cross-cultural adaptation into the German language. *Nervenarzt* 2010;980-985.

18 Soh SE, Morris ME, McGinley JL. Determinants of health-related quality of life in Parkinson's disease: A systematic review. *Parkinsonism Relat Disord* 2011;17:1-9.

19 Martinez-Martin P, Schapira AH, Stocchi F, et al. Prevalence of nonmotor symptoms in Parkinson's disease in an international setting; study using nonmotor symptoms questionnaire in 545 patients. *Mov Disord* 2007;22:1623-1629.

20 Honig H, Antonini A, Martinez-Martin P, et al. Intrajejunal levodopa infusion in Parkinson's disease: a pilot multicenter study of effects on nonmotor symptoms and quality of life. *Mov Disord* 2009;24:1468-1474.

21 Evatt ML, Chaudhuri KR, Chour KL, et al. Dysautonomia rating scales in Parkinson's disease: sialorrhea, dysphagia, and constipation – critique and recommendations by movement disorders task force on rating scales for Parkinson's disease. *Mov Disord* 2009;24:635-646.

22 Simkin S, Chaudhuri KR, Selway N. Subthalmic nucleus (STN) deep brain stimulation (DBS) and the non-motor symptom scale (NMSS) in Parkinson's disease (PD). *Mov Disord* 2006;21:S685.

23 Kim HJ, Park SY, Cho YJ, et al. Nonmotor symptoms in de novo Parkinson disease before and after dopaminergic treatment. *J Neurol* Sci 2009;287:200-204.

24 Braak H, Del Tredici K, Rub U, De Vos RA, Jansen Steur EN, Braak E. Staging of brain pathology related to sporadic Parkinson's disease. *Neurobiol Aging* 2003;24:197-211.

25 Tolosa E, Compta Y, Gaig C. The premotor phase of Parkinson's disease. *Parkinsonism Relat Disord* 2007;13:S2-S7.

26 Parkinson Study Group. Dopamine transporter brain imaging to assess the effects of pramipexole vs levodopa on Parkinson disease progression. *JAMA* 2002;287:1653-1661.

27 Parkinson Study Group. A controlled, randomized, delayed-start study of rasagiline in early Parkinson disease. *Arch Neurol* 2004;61:561-566.

28 Whone AL, Watts RL, Stoessl AJ, et al. Slower progression of Parkinson's disease with ropinirole versus levodopa: The REAL-PET study. *Ann Neurol* 2003;54:93-101.

29 Olanow CW, Rascol O, Hauser RE, et al. A double-blind, delayed-start trial of rasagiline in Parkinson's disease. *N Engl J Med* 2009;361:1268-1278.

30 De La Fuente-Fernandez R, Schulzer M, Mak E, Sossi V. Trials of neuroprotective therapies for Parkinson's disease: Problems and limitations. *Parkinsonism Relat Disord* 2010;16:365-369.

Chapter 5

Neuropsychiatric symptoms

Per Odin and Kerstin Dietrich

Neuropsychiatric problems represent a major group of non-motor symptoms (NMSs) that require effective management. They can range from depression, anxiety, compulsive disorders and hallucinations to dementia, so they are a significant cause of disability and reduced health-related quality of life (HRQoL) for affected patients, and also substantially increase distress to caregivers [1]. It has been found that non-tremor-dominant Parkinson's disease (PD) is associated with an increased risk of cognitive deterioration, depression, apathy and hallucinations compared with other motor subtypes of PD [2].

Apathy

Apathy is a specific symptom of PD, which might occur together with or separately from depression [3]. Apathy seems to be independent of somnolence and fatigue [4,5], but it might coexist with anxiety problems. Patients with PD more frequently have apathy compared with other chronic diseases, which can indicate a neurodegenerative origin [6]. Apathy might be related to dopaminergic deficits in some cases, but in other situations it can be unresponsive to dopaminergic therapy. There are reports of dopamine agonists improving apathy in some patients with PD [7]. Another study showed that levodopa treatment could reverse apathy in the 'on' stage compared with the 'off' stage [8]. However, other

K. R. Chaudhuri et al., *Handbook of Non-Motor Symptoms in Parkinson's Disease*, DOI: 10.1007/978-1-908517-60-9_5, © Springer Healthcare, a part of Springer Science+Business Media 2011

studies have postulated that apathy can be unresponsive to dopaminergic therapy [9] and involvement of other neurotransmitter pathways than the dopaminergic ones is likely [10]. The RECOVER study reported a significant ($p<0.001$) improvement on two items related to apathy in the NMSS with rotigotine patch but not placebo. This would suggest further studies addressing treatment of apathy using longer acting dopamine agonists may be warranted [11].

Depression

Depression is an important neuropsychiatric symptom in PD. There is a strong correlation between depression and HRQoL. Clinically relevant depressive symptoms occur in up to 45% of PD patients [9]. The depression is characterized by a feeling of guilt, lack of self-esteem, sadness and remorse. Depression can precede the development of PD and there is no correlation with the severity of motor impairment. One study reported that depressed patients are more likely to develop PD than osteoarthritis or diabetes patients [12]. A retrospective cohort study showed that, at the time of diagnosis of PD, 9.2% of the patients had a lifetime diagnosis of depression compared with 4.2% in the control group. Although suicidal ideation occurs in PD patients, deaths by suicide are rare, with the possible exception of patients who have had their dopaminergic drugs withdrawn or reduced too quickly after undergoing subthalamic nucleus stimulation [13,14].

Due to the overlap with other NMSs and the fact that the core symptoms of depression such as anhedonia, anergia, decreased concentration and sleep disturbances can often be difficult to distinguish from PD, diagnosis can be difficult and the condition is often under-diagnosed [15]. Therefore more than 50% of all PD patients do not receive treatment for depression [16]. One proposed reason for this statistic is that physicians often think that the depression is reactive to the motor impairment. However, a significant biological rather than a purely reactive basis is probable. Dysfunction of dopaminergic, serotoninergic and noradrenergic pathways in the limbic system has been implicated [17].

Depression rating scales, such as the Beck Depression Inventory, Hamilton Depression Rating Scale and Montgomery Asberg Depression

Rating Scale, have been used as screening tools for depression in PD, although they are not specific for PD [18]. Therefore a depression scale specific for PD is required and work is in progress.

There have been many attempts to use dopaminergic therapies, including levodopa and dopamine agonists, for the treatment of depression in PD. In particular, pramipexole, but also ropinirole and pergolide, have shown capacity to improve depression [19–24]. The recently published RECOVER study examined the effect of the rotigotine patch on early morning motor function and sleep in PD with effect on non-motor symptoms such as depression as secondary outcome variables. A statistically significant improvement in depression scores measured by the Beck Depression Inventory as well as the depression sub-domain of the NMSS was recorded, with rotigotine and not placebo further emphasising the role of targeted dopamine agonist treatment for depression in PD [25].

The published evidence regarding treatment options for depression in PD is very limited. There is a profound need for systematic controlled studies. At the same time it is evident that there are treatment options. As a result of the strong influence of depression on HRQoL it is important to detect and treat depression in PD. The first step should be to optimize the dopaminergic treatment. In this context the dopamine agonists might be of special interest because of the evidence for antidepressant effects. Among the antidepressant drugs, both the old tricyclic antidepressants [26–28] and the newer selective serotonin reuptake inhibitors (SSRIs) and serotonin–noradrenaline reuptake inhibitors (SNRIs) [29] can be considered. As a result of the favorable side-effect profile, the newer compounds should be considered as first-line therapy, especially in the older patient groups – in spite of having less evidence for effect than tricyclic antidepressants. So-called 'new' antidepressants, such as mirtazapine, reboxetine and venlafaxine, can also be considered (although very little evidence has been published to date).

Anxiety

Anxiety disorders are very common in PD and can occur before motor symptoms [30,31]. The prevalence is 25–40% [32] and therefore higher than in other chronic diseases. Anxiety can present as panic attacks, phobias or generalized anxiety disorder. It might be the result of specific neurobiological and neuropeptide abnormalities associated with PD [33] and, as it is frequently associated with depression, the same pathophysiology has been implicated [34]. From a clinical point of view many symptoms of anxiety, including panic attacks, breathlessness, restlessness and dizziness, can occur as a dopamine-deficit event as part of an 'off' period [34]. In this case, the anxiety improves with an improved dopaminergic therapy, with less 'off' time. Similarly, anxiety related to depression often responds to dopaminergic therapy. On the other hand, there are forms of anxiety, such as the fear of dying or going insane, that are independent of dopaminergic state and that do not respond to improvement of the dopaminergic therapy; these may be more likely to be reactive symptoms to the diagnosis and progressive PD symptomatology [32]. Occasionally anxiety syndromes and mania have been reported as side effects of dopamine agonist treatment and high-dose levodopa treatment [35].

When treating anxiety in PD, the first step is to optimize the dopaminergic therapy [36,37]. Other types of medication that have been used in this connection are SNRIs, SSRIs and tricyclic antidepressants. Further benzodiazepines and pregabaline have been suggested as effective. There is, however, limited evidence for effect, so far.

Attention and memory

Cognitive dysfunction is common in patients with advanced PD. However, cognitive problems can also occur in early stages of the disease. They then often present as a frontal dysexecutive syndrome, with difficulties in maintaining an adaptive response against competing alternatives [38]. Some patients can also have visuospatial or visuoperceptual deficits [39]. An investigation on patients with early PD showed that 57% had mild cognitive impairment [40]. The early cognitive changes in PD might involve the caudate and corticostriatal pathways [41]. Abnormal dopamine uptake and abnormal brain metabolism in cortical targets for dopaminergic fibers have been described [42,43]. There are indications that at least some aspects of the cognitive dysfunction might improve with dopaminergic therapy [44,45]. Dopaminergic treatment might, however, also worsen cognitive functions, particularly in patients with advanced disease.

Hallucinations, delusions and psychosis

Psychosis is one of the most disabling non-motor complications of PD. Psychotic symptoms strongly correlate with the need for nursing home placement and with mortality [46,47]. Visual hallucinations have been observed in up to 40% of patients with advanced disease [46,48]. These visual hallucinations range from passing shadows in the periphery (de passage hallucinations) and misinterpretation of objects to vivid recognizable people or animals [49]. In most cases such hallucinations are benign, and in time become recognized and disregarded in patients [49], but there is a tendency to develop more severe symptoms such as delusions, paranoid ideation and delirium, and for this to become more frequent in most patients. Occasionally auditory hallucinations also appear; this can, however, be a sign of depression. Although visual hallucinations are often regarded as side effects of medication, neuronal degeneration of the pedunculopontine nucleus, locus ceruleus and dopaminergic raphe nuclei can be causative [50]. These nuclei are also involved in causation of rapid eye movement (REM) sleep behavior disorder, which has been suggested as a risk factor for hallucinations [51].

Visual hallucinations often precede or accompany cognitive decline and should be considered as a warning sign for developing dementia in PD. Age, duration of disease and depression are probably not implicated [46]. A hypothesis behind the development of psychiatric symptoms is that psychosis starts with drug-induced sleep disruption, which leads to vivid dreams, hallucinations and delirium [52]. Genetic risk factors have also been suggested and a polymorphism in the cholecystokinin gene could be involved [53]. Delusions are less frequent than hallucinations, but can be upsetting for caregivers and relatives because they are frequently paranoid or accusatory in nature, often involving suspicions of spousal infidelity or abandonment [31].

Delirium can occur in advanced dementia and can be precipitated by concurrent infection or dopaminergic drugs. Sudden withdrawal of dopaminergic drugs can induce neuroleptic malignant syndrome, which may be associated with delirium [54].

Psychosis typically begins 10 years after diagnosis of PD and earlier onset suggests an alternative diagnosis such as Alzheimer's disease,

Lewy body dementia, or a previous history of psychosis [55]. Imaging results have shown higher concentrations of Lewy bodies in the para-hippocampus, amygdala, and frontal, temporal and parietal lobes in PD patients with psychosis [31]. Currently, there is no specific tool for assessing delusions, hallucinations and psychoses in PD patients. The Parkinson's Psychosis Rating Scale (PPRS), the NMSQuest and the SCales for Outcomes in PArkinson's disease – Psychosocial question-naire (SCOPA-PS) cover hallucinations in some sub-items only. A recent 20-item questionnaire called the University of Miami Parkinson's Disease Hallucinations Questionnaire (UM-PDHQ) demonstrated the key char-acteristics of hallucinations in detail but it has not yet been validated in large population studies [56].

Due to the prominent role of dopaminergic treatment in inducing psychosis in PD, interventions are based first of all on reduction or withdrawal of the offending drugs, complemented by adjunct treatment with atypical antipsychotics. However, infection and metabolic disorders can provoke psychosis and, in such cases, the underlying disorder should be treated. The first step is normally to control triggering factors, including treatment of infections and metabolic disorders, normalizing fluid/electrolyte balance and treating sleep disturbance. The next step should be to exclude drugs that might have negative effects such as anticholinergics, antidepressants, phenothiazines and uro-spasmolytics. The third step should be to reduce anti-parkinsonian therapy, first stopping anticholinergics, then amantadine, dopamine agonists, monoamine oxidase B (MAO-B) inhibitors, and lastly catechol-O-methyltransferase (COMT) inhibitors and levodopa. This is therefore a change towards monotherapy with levodopa. As a next step atypical neuroleptics can be added; clozapine has best evidence of effect [57,58], but it has a potential risk for haematological side effects and blood must be monitored. Quetiapine is probably also useful [59–67], even if evidence for this is non-consistent. Quetiapine is relatively safe and blood monitoring is not necessary. All other neuroleptic drugs can worsen the PD symptomatology and are potentially dangerous. A further option is to add cholinesterase inhibitors, either rivastigmine [68–70] or donepezil [71,72].

Compulsive behaviors

Compulsive behaviors can include a variety of actions, from pathological shopping, eating, collecting, gambling and sexual preoccupations, to medication abuse [73]. These behaviors are problematic not only for the patient but also for the caregiver and are often not declared because they may be socially unacceptable, embarrassing and a source of financial distress. Therefore, physicians must specifically ask for the presence of these behaviors. Their overall occurrence appears to be approximately 6% of treated PD patients, with pathological gambling ranging between 3% and 8%, hypersexuality occurring in 2–8% and compulsive medication use probably of lower frequency – 3% or 4% [73]. Dopamine agonist (DA) use has a greater association with these behaviors than levodopa, as does being young and male [74], so a fine balancing act must be achieved when using dopamine agonists. Alterations in dopaminergic functions within the nucleus accumbens and ventral striatum is the proposed pathophysiology, in line with data on addiction [75]. Levodopa is mainly implicated in dopamine dysregulation syndrome, associated with medication overuse and a scenario similar to substance abuse.

Dopamine agonist withdrawal syndrome

Another spectrum is the recently described dopamine agonist withdrawal syndrome, which is related to sudden or rapid stoppage of dopamine agonists in patients suspected of suffering from impulse control disorders [76]. This condition resembles neuroleptic malignant syndrome in extreme cases and therefore, in cases where such a strategy is contemplated, slow or gradual reduction of agonists is recommended.

Cognitive dysfunction and dementia

The point prevalence of dementia in PD is 30–40% [77]; the cumulative incidence is closer to 80% [78]. It has been estimated that PD-associated dementia accounts for at least 3% or 4% of dementia in the general population [79]. PD patients have a fivefold increased risk of developing dementia than their equivalent non-affected age group [80]. High rates of dementia have been reported by Hely and colleagues [81], among others, in a 15- to 18-year follow-up of patients with PD. Current age, rather than disease duration, is the main risk factor for development of dementia [82]; other risk factors include familial dementia, severe extrapyramidal symptoms, low educational level, and psychosis or confusion after levodopa medication [83]. The dementia is progressive and clinically characterized by a dysexecutive syndrome with impairment of visuospatial functions and memory and disorientation [83]. Often there is a loss of response to treatment with dopaminergic drugs in parallel. Degeneration of nigral cells probably plays a role.

Cortical and subcortical Lewy bodies are also thought to be causative, even if this is more controversial [84,85]. Cholinergic cell loss in the nucleus basalis of Meynert is pronounced and forms a rational for cholinergic treatment of dementia in PD. A contribution of a parallel Alzheimer pathology, as well as vascular pathology and genetic factors, has been suggested [86]. Interestingly, it has been found that cognitive decline is correlated to PD subtype; PD-associated dementia did not occur in patients with tremor-dominant PD [83].

With regard to treatment of dementia in PD, the first step should be to discontinue drugs that can aggravate cognitive difficulties. This includes anticholinergics, amantadine, tricyclic antidepressants, tolterodine, oxybutynin and benzodiazepines. The next step is to add cholinesterase inhibitors. Evidence is available for the effect of rivastigmine [69] and donepezil [87–89]. The effects of galantamine are less well documented [90]. Memantine can be considered as an addition or alternative [91–92].

References

1   Löhle M, Storch A, Reichmann H. Beyond tremor and rigidity: non-motor features of Parkinson's disease. *J Neural Transm* 2009;116:1483-1492.
2   Reijnders J, Ehrt U, Lousberg R, Aarsland D, Leentjens A. The association between motor subtypes and psychopathology in Parkinson's disease. *Parkinsonism Relat Disord* 2009;15:379-382.
3   Oguru M, Tachibana H, Toda K, Okuda B, Oka N. Apathy and depression in Parkinson's disease. *J Geriatr Psychiatry Neurol* 2010;23:35-41.
4   Starkstein SE, Mayberg SE, Prezioso TJ, et al. Reliability, validity, and clinical correlates of apathy in Parkinson's disease. *J Neuropsychiatry* 1992;4:134-139.
5   Pluck GC, Brown RG. Apathy in Parkinson's disease. *J Neurol Neurosurg Psychiatry* 2002;73:636-642.
6   Alves G, Wentzel-Larsen T, Jansen JP. Is fatigue and independent and persistent symptom in patients with Parkinson's disease? *Neurology* 2004;63:1908-1911.
7   Czernecki V, Pillon B, Houeto JL, et al. Motivation, reward and Parkinson's disease: influence of L-dopa therapy. *Neuropsychologia* 2002;40:2257-2267.
8   Marin RS, Fogel BS, Hawkin J, et al. Apathy: a treatable syndrome. *J Neuropsychiatry Clin Neurosci* 1995;7:23-30.

9 Chaudhuri K, Schapira A. Non-motor symptoms of Parkinson's disease: dopaminergic pathophysiology and treatment. *Lancet Neurol* 2009;8:464-474.

10 Brown RG, Pluck G. Negative symptoms: the 'pathology' of motivation and goal-directed behavior. *Trends Neurosci* 2000;23:412-417.

11 Chaudhuri KR, Joseph H. Friedman, Erwin Surmann, et al; on behalf of the RECOVER study investigators. The effects of transdermal rotigotine on mood/cognition: interpretations from a post hoc analysis of the RECOVER Study using the Parkinson's disease Non-Motor Symptom Scale. Poster presented at: 15th International Congress of Parkinson's Disease and Movement Disorders; June 5-9, 2011; Toronto, Canada.

12 Nilsson FM, Kessig LV, Bolwig TG. Increased risk of developing Parkinson's disease for patients with major affective disorders. *Acta Psychiatr Scand* 2001;104:380-386.

13 Myslobodsky M, Lalonde FM, Hicks L. Are patients with Parkinson's disease suicidal? *J Geriatr Psychiatry Neurol* 2001;14:120-124.

14 Funkiewiez A, Ardouin C, Caputo E, et al. Long-term effects of bilateral subthalamic nucleus stimulation on cognitive function, mood, and behavior in Parkinson's disease. *J Neurol Neurosurg Psychiatry* 2004;75:834-839.

15 Reichmann H, Schneider C, Löhle M. Non-motor features of Parkinson's disease: depression and dementia. *Parkinsonism Relat Disord* 2009;15:S87-S92.

16 Shulman L. Non-recognition of depression and other non-motor symptoms in Parkinson's disease. *Parkinsonism Relat Disord* 2002;8:193-197.

17 Remy P, Doder M, Lees A, et al. Depression in Parkinson's disease. Loss of dopamine and noradrenaline innervations in the limbic system. *Brain* 2005;128:1314-1322.

18 Miyasaki J, Shannon K, Voon V, Ravina B, Kleiner-Fisman G, Anderson K. Practice parameter: evaluation and treatment of depression, psychosis, and dementia in Parkinson disease (an evidence-based review): report of the Quality Standards Subcommittee of the American Academy of Neurology. *Neurology* 2006;66:996-1002.

19 Corrigan M, Denahan AQ, Wright CE, et al. Comparison of pramipexole and placebo in patients with major depression. *Depress Anxiety* 2000;11: 58-65.

20 Reichmann H, Brech MH, Koster J. Pramipexole in routine clinical practice: a prospective observational trial in Parkinson's disease. *CNS Drugs* 2003;17:965-973.

21 Rektorova I, Rektor I, Bares M, et al. Pramipexole and pergolide in the treatment of depression in Parkinson's disease: a national multicentre prospective randomized study. *Eur J Neurol* 2003;10:399-406.

22 Goldberg J, Burdick KE, Endick CJ. Preliminary randomized placebo controlled trial to pramipexole added to mood stabilizers for treatment of resistant bipolar depression. *Am J Psychiatry* 2004;161:564-566.

23 Barone P, Scarzella L, Marconi R, et al. Pramipexole versus sertraline in the treatment of depression in Parkinson's disease. A national multicenter parallel group randomized study. *J Neurol* 2006;253:601-607.

24 Pahwa R, Stacy MA, Factor SA, et al; on behalf of the EASE-PD adjunct study investigators. Ropinirole 24-hour prolonged release: randomized controlled study in advanced Parkinson's disease. *Neurology* 2007; 68:1108-1115.

25 Trenkwalder C, Kies B, Rudzinska M, et al, and the RECOVER study group. Rotigotine effects on early morning motor function and sleep in Parkinson's disease: A double-blind, randomised, placebo-controlled study (RECOVER). Mov Disord 2011;26:90-99.

26 Ghazi-Noori S, Chung TH, Deane KHO, Rickards H, Clarke CE. Therapies for depression in Parkinson's disease. *Cochrane Database Syst Rev* 2003;2:CD003465.

27 Menza M, Dobkin RD, Marin H, et al. The impact of treatment of depression on quality of life, disability and relapse in patients with Parkinson's disease. *Mov Disord* 2009;24:1325-1332.

28 Menza M, Dobkin R, Marin H, et al. A controlled trial of antidepressants in patients with Parkinson disease and depression. *Neurology* 2009;72:886-892.

29 Weintraub D, Morales KH, Moberg PJ, et al. Antidepressant studies in Parkinson's disease: a review and meta-analysis. *Mov Disord* 2005;20:1161-1169.

30 Shiba M, Bower JH, Maragonare DM, et al. Anxiety disorders and depressive disorders preceding Parkinson's disease: a case-control study. *Mov Disord* 2000;15:669-677.

31 Weisskopf MG, Chen H, Schwarzschild MA, Kawachi I, Ascherio A. Prospective study of phobic anxiety and risk of Parkinson's disease. *Mov Disord* 2003;18:646-651.

32 Park A, Stacy M. Non-motor symptoms in Parkinson's disease. *J Neurol* 2009;256:293-298.

33 Richard IH, Schiffer RB, Kurlan R. Anxiety and Parkinson's disease. *J Neuropsychiatry Clin Neurosci* 1996;8:383-392.

34 Goetz C. New developments in depression, anxiety, compulsiveness, and hallucinations in Parkinson's disease. *Mov Disord* 2010;25:S104-S109.

35 Singh A, Althoff R, Martineau J, Jacobson J. Pramipexole, ropinirole and mania in Parkinson's disease. *Am J Psychiatry* 2005;162:814-815.

36 Witjas T, Kaphan E, Regis J, et al. Effects of chronic subthalamic stimulation on nonmotor fluctuations in Parkinson's disease. *Mov Disord* 2007;22:1729-1734.

37 Witt K, Daniels C, Reiff J, et al. Neuropsychological and psychiatric changes after deep brain stimulation for Parkinson's disease: a randomised, multicentre study. *Lancet Neurol* 2008;7:605-614.

38 Dubois B, Pillon B. Cognitive deficits in Parkinson's disease. *J Neurol* 1997;244:2–8.

39 Uc E, Rizzo M, Anderson S, Qian S, Rodnitzky R, Dawson J. Visual dysfunction in Parkinson's disease without dementia. *Neurology* 2005;65:1907-1913.

40 Williams-Gray C, Foltynie T, Brayne C, Robbins T, Barker R. Evolution of cognitive dysfunction in and incident Parkinson's disease cohort. *Parkinsonism Relat Disord* 2007;13:1787-1798.

41 Emre M. What causes mental dysfunction in Parkinson's disease? *Mov Disord* 2003a;18:S63-S71.

42 Rinne J, Portin R, Ruottinen H, et al. Cognitive impairment and the brain dopaminergic system in Parkinson disease – F18 fluorodopa positron emission tomographic study. *Arch Neurol* 2000;57:470-475.

43 Lewis S, Dove A, Robbins T, Barker R, Owen A. Cognitive impairments in early Parkinson's disease are accompanied by reductions in activity in frontostriatal neural circuitry. *J Neurosci* 2003;23:6351-6356.

44 Cools R, Stefanova E, Barker R, Robbins T, Owen A. Dopaminergic modulation of high-level cognition in Parkinson's disease: the role of the prefrontal cortex revealed by PET. *Brain* 2002;125:584-594.

45 Mattay V, Tessitore A, Callicott J, et al. Dopaminergic modulation of cortical function in patients with Parkinson's disease. *Ann Neurol* 2002;51:156-164.

46 Aarsland D, Larsen J, Tandber E, Laake K. Predictors of nursing home placement in Parkinson's disease: a population-based, prospective study. *J Am Geriatr Soc* 2000;48:938-942.

47 Fenelon G, Mahieux F, Huon R, et al. Hallucinations in Parkinson's disease: prevalence, phenomenology, and risk factors. *Brain* 2000;123:733-745.

48 Papapetropoulos S, Mash D. Psychotic symptoms in Parkinson's disease. From description to etiology. *J Neurol* 2005;252:753-764.

49 Diederich N, Pieri V, Goetz C. Coping strategies for visual hallucinations in Parkinson's disease. *Mov Disord* 2003;18:831-832.

50 Diederich NJ, Goetz CG, Stebbins GT. Repeated visual hallucinations in Parkinson's disease as disturbed external/internal perceptions: focused review and new integrative model. *Mov Disord* 2005;20:130-140.

51 Onofrj M, Thomas A, D'Andreamatteo G, et al. Incidence of RBD and hallucination in patients affected by Parkinson's disease: 8 year follow-up. *Neuro Sci* 2002;23:S91-S94.

52 Moskovitz C, Moses H, Klawans HL. Levodopa-induced psychosis: a kindling phenomenon. *Am J Psychiatry* 1978;135:669-675.

53 Goldman JG, Goetz CG, Berry-Kravis E, Leurgans S, Zhou L. Genetic polymorphisms in Parkinson's disease subjects with and without hallucinations: an analysis of the cholecystokinin system. *Arch Neurol* 2004;61:1280-1284.

54 Kipps CM, Fung VSC, Grattan-Smith P, de Moore GM, Morris JGL. Movement disorder emergencies. *Mov Disord* 2005;20:322-334.

55 Fenelon G. Psychosis in Parkinson's disease: phenomenology, frequency, risk factors, and current understanding of pathophysiologic mechanisms. *CNS Spectr* 2008;13:18-25.

56 Papapetropoulos S, Katzen H, Schrag A., Singer C, Scanlon B, Nation D. A questionnaire-based (UM-PDHQ) study of hallucinations in Parkinson's disease. *BMC Neurol* 2008;8:21.

57 Parkinson Study Group. Low-dose clozapine for the treatment of drug-induced psychosis in Parkinson's disease. *N Engl J Med* 1999;340:757-763.

58 French Clozapine Parkinson Study Group. Clozapine in drug-induced psychosis in Parkinson's disease. *Lancet* 1999;353:2041.

59 Fernandez H, Friedman J, Jacques C, Rosenfeld M. Quetiapine for the treatment of drug-induced psychosis in Parkinson's disease. *Mov Disord* 1999;14:484-487.

60 Fernandez H, Trieschmann ME, Burke MA, Friedmann JH. Quetiapine for psychosis in Parkinson's disease versus dementia with Lewy bodies. *J Clin Psychiatry* 2002;63:513-515.

61 Fernandez HH, Trieschmann ME, Burke MA, Jacques C, Friedman JH. Long-term outcome of quetiapine use for psychosis among Parkinsonian patients. *Mov Disord* 2003;18:510-514.

62 Dewey RB Jr, O'Suilleabhain PE. Treatment of drug-induced psychosis with quetiapine and clozapine in Parkinson's disease. *Neurology* 2000;55:1753-1754.

63 Brandstaedter D, Oertel WH. Treatment of drug-induced psychosis with quetiapine and clozapine in Parkinson's disease. *Neurology* 2002;58:160-161.

64 Reddy S, Factor SA, Molho ES, Feustel PJ. The effect of quetiapine on psychosis and motor function in parkinsonian patients with and without dementia. *Mov Disord* 2002;17:676-681.

65 Juncos JL, Roberts VJ, Evatt ML, et al. Quetiapine improves psychotic symptoms and cognition in Parkinson's disease. *Mov Disord* 2004;19:29-35.

66 Morgante L, Epifanio A, Spina E, et al. Quetiapine and clozapine in parkinsonian patients with dopaminergic psychosis. *Clin Neuropharmacol* 2004;27:153-156.

67 Ondo WG, Tintner R, Voung KD, Lai D, Ringholz G. Double-blind, placebo-controlled, unforced titration parallel trial of quetiapine for dopaminergic-induced hallucinations in Parkinson's disease. *Mov Disord* 2005;20:958-963.

68 Bullock R, Cameron A. Rivastigmine for the treatment of dementia and visual hallucinations associated with Parkinson's disease: a case series. *Curr Med Res Opin* 2002;18:258-264.

69 Emre M, Aarsland D, Albanese A, et al. Rivastigmine in Parkinson's disease patients with dementia: a randomized, double-blind, placebo-controlled study. *N Engl J Med* 2004;351:2509-2518.

70 Burn D, Emre M, McKeith I, et al. Effects of rivastigmine in patients with and without visual hallucinations in dementia associated with Parkinson's disease. *Mov Disord* 2006;21:1899-1907.

71 Bergmann J, Lerner V. Successful use of donepezil for the treatment of psychotic symptoms in patients with Parkinson's disease. *Clin Neuropharmacol* 2002;25:107-110.

72 Fabbrini G, Barbanti P, Aurilia C, Pauletti C, Lenzi GL, Meco G. Donepezil in the treatment of hallucinations and delusions in Parkinson's disease. *Neurol Sci* 2002;23:41-43.

73 Voon V, Potenza M, Thomsen T. Medication-induced impulse control and repetitive behaviors in Parkinson's disease. *Curr Opin Neurol* 2007;20:484-442.

74 Weintraub D. Impulse control disorders in Parkinson's disease: prevalence and possible risk factors. *Parkinsonism Relat Disord* 2009;15:S110-S113.

75 Evans A, Pavese N, Lawrence A. Compulsive drug use linked to sensitized ventral striatal dopamine transmission. *Ann Neurol* 2006;59:852-858.

76 Rabinak CA, Koester J, Potenza MN, et al. Dopamine agonist withdrawal syndrome in Parkinson's disease. *Arch Neurol* 2010;67:58-63.

77 Aarsland D, Zaccai J, Brayne C. A systematic review of prevalence studies of dementia in Parkinson's disease. *Mov Disord* 2005;20:1255-1263.

78 Aarsland D, Andersen K, Larsen JP, Lolk A, Kragh-Sorensen P. Prevalence and characteristics of dementia in Parkinson disease: an 8-year prospective study. *Arch Neurol* 2003;60:387-392.

79 Hobson P, Meara J. Risk and incidence of dementia in a cohort of older subjects with Parkinson's disease in the United Kingdom. *Mov Disord* 2004;19:1043-1049.

80 Emre M. Dementia associated with Parkinson's disease. *Lancet Neurol* 2003b;2:229-237.

81 Hely MA, Morris JGL, Reid WGJ, Trafficante R. Sydney multicenter study on Parkinson's disease: non-L-dopa-responsive problems dominate at 15 years. *Mov Disord* 2005;20:190-199.

82 Buter TC, van den Hout A, Matthews FE, Larsen JP, Brayne C, Aarsland D. Dementia and survival in Parkinson disease: a 12-year population study. *Neurology* 2008;70:1017-1022.

83 Ziemssen T, Reichmann H. Non-motor dysfunction in Parkinson's disease. *Parkinsonism Relat Disord* 2007;13:323-332.

84 Mattila PM, Rinne JO, Helenius H, Dickson DW, Röyttä M. Alpha-synuclein-immunoreative cortical Lewy bodies are associated with cognitive impairment in Parkinson's disease. *Acta Neuropathol* 2000;100:285-290.

85 Cummings J. Reconsidering diagnostic criteria for dementia with Lewy bodies: highlights from the Third International Workshop on Dementia with Lewy bodies and Parkinson's disease dementia, September 17–20, 2003, Newcastle upon Tyne, UK. *Rev Neurol Dis* 2004;1:31-34.

86 Li YJ, Hauser MA, Scott WK, et al. Apolipoprotein E controls the risk and age at onset of Parkinson's disease. *Neurology* 2004;62:2005-2009.

87 Aarsland D, Laake K, Larsen JP, Janvin C. Donepezil for cognitive impairment in Parkinson's disease: a randomised controlled study. *J Neurol Neurosurg Psychiatry* 2002;72:708-712.

88 Leroi I, Brandt J, Reich SG, Lyketsos CG, Grill S, Thompson R, Marsh L. Randomized placebocontrolled trial of donepezil in cognitive impairment in Parkinson's disease. *Int J Geriatr Psychiatry* 2004;19:1-8.

89 Ravina B, Putt M, Siderowf A, et al. Donepezil for dementia in Parkinson's disease: a randomised, double blind, placebo controlled, crossover study. *J Neurol Neurosurg Psychiatry* 2005;76:934-939.

90 Litvinenko IV, Odinak MM, Mogil'naya VI, Emelin AY. Efficacy and safety of galantamine (Reminyl) for dementia in patients with Parkinson's disease (an open controlled trial). *Neurosci Behav Physiol* 2008;38:937-945.

91 Aarsland D, Ballard C, Walker Z, et al. Memantine in patients with Parkinson's disease dementia or dementia with Lewy bodies: a double-blind, placebo-controlled, multicentre trial. *Lancet Neurol* 2009;8:613-618.

92 Leroi I, Overshott R, Byrne EJ, Daniel E, Burns A. Randomized controlled trial of memantine in dementia associated with Parkinson's disease. *Mov Disord* 2009;24:1217-1221.

Chapter 6

Sleep-related symptoms

Per Odin

Nocturnal non-motor symptoms

Nearly all Parkinson's disease (PD) patients have sleep disturbances that usually start early in the disease onset, with studies indicating a prevalence of 60–98% [1–3]. The more common are rapid eye movement (REM), sleep behavior disorder (RBD), insomnia, nightmares, snoring, restless legs syndrome (RLS) and sleep ambulism. The pathogenesis of sleep disruption is multifactorial, but degeneration of central sleep regulation centers in the brain stem and thalamocortical pathways is likely to be important. The pedunculopontine nucleus, locus ceruleus and retrorubral nucleus influence normal REM atonia and phasic generator circuitry, and have been implicated in the pathogenesis of RBD [4,5]. Other factors that may contribute to sleep disruption include motor symptoms, anxiety, depression and dopaminergic treatment. Some non-motor symptoms (NMSs) cause abnormalities in the primary sleep architecture and have a secondary effect on quality of sleep, such as nocturia. Sleep disorder breathing due to obstructive sleep apnea, not necessarily associated with obesity, and a narcoleptic pattern of rapid-onset sleep are also important causes of sleep-related morbidity in PD [1,6].

Sleep disorders in PD can be easily recognized and quantified during consultations using validated rating instruments, such as the Epworth Sleepiness Scale (ESS) and the Pittsburgh Sleep Quality Index (PSQI), or

K. R. Chaudhuri et al., *Handbook of Non-Motor Symptoms in Parkinson's Disease*, DOI: 10.1007/978-1-908517-60-9_6,
© Springer Healthcare, a part of Springer Science+Business Media 2011

by PD-specific assessment tools such as the Non-Motor Symptom Scale (NMSS), Parkinson's Disease Sleep Scale (PDSS and PDSS-2) or the SCales for Outcomes in PArkinson's disease – Sleep (SCOPA-S) questionnaire [7]. Furthermore, polysomnography (PSG) and multiple sleep latency tests can be used to verify preliminary diagnoses. A recent clinical trial has shown that melatonin improves the symptoms of RBD [8] and may be a second useful agent for this disorder besides clonazepam.

Restless legs syndrome and periodic limb movements

Periodic limb movements and restless legs syndrome (RLS) are closely linked and are sensitive to dopaminergic treatment [9,10], with 61% of PD patients reporting that RLS onset correlated with 'wearing off' at night [11]. RLS is defined as an unpleasant feeling in a limb that appears or worsens when a person is sitting or lying still, mainly in the evening or night, and is relieved with movement for at least as long as the activity continues [12]. The relationship between PD and RLS is still not completely clear [13] and because of overlapping symptomatology it is often difficult to estimate whether RLS is present in PD patients. Several studies have reported an increased prevalence of RLS in PD, and periodic limb movements are another frequent cause of sleep disruption [13–15]. The prevalence of restless legs in PD is estimated at 20%, compared with around 10% in the general population. A recent study found that, within the study population, RLS symptom onset was around 4.5 years (± 3.7 years) after PD onset [11], but the symptoms of RLS can appear before those of PD, and RLS patients in general do not have a higher risk of developing PD compared with non-RLS patients [11,14].

The pathophysiology of RLS and periodic limb movements is thought to be related to changes in mesocortical dopamine; in this it is distinct from PD pathology, which involves deterioration of the nigrostriatal pathway [12].

There are very few trials exploring the effect of dopaminergic medication in patients with PD and RLS. One small placebo-controlled trial reported that continuous infusion of apomorphine, a non-ergot dopamine agonist, given subcutaneously overnight, resulted in significantly reduced nocturnal discomfort, decreased leg movements, and improved pain and spasm scores in six patients [16]. An open-label study of 15 patients with PD and periodic limb movements, who received cabergoline, reported reduced periodic limb movements in sleep, although there were increased numbers of awakenings and stage shifts [17]. The quality standards subcommittee of the American Academy of Neurology (AAN) concluded that there is evidence that levodopa improves periodic limb movement in the night [18]. For dopamine agonists, the committee found that the evidence for effect was insufficient. In a practical clinical setting, restless legs in PD can be treated as restless legs in general; serum ferritin can be analyzed and if indicated iron treatment can be given (parenteral treatment should be considered in case of parallel treatment with levodopa to avoid interaction). If pharmacological treatment is necessary, long-acting dopamine agonists can be considered in the evening, and, if necessary, combined with levodopa. In some cases opioids (tramadol, codeine), anti-epileptics (gabapentin) and benzodiazepines (clonazepam) can also be considered.

Insomnia

Difficulty falling asleep and difficulties maintaining sleep are both common in PD [19]. Sleep-maintenance problems can be caused by many different problems, such as night-time akinesia, off-state motor and non-motor problems, such as nocturia, RLS, periodic limb movements and reversal of sleep patterns [1,20]. In a double-blind, placebo-controlled trial in elderly PD patients, it was shown that levodopa/carbidopa tablets before sleep could improve sleep quality and early morning walking [21]. In another study it was shown that slow-release levodopa at bedtime did improve night-time akinesia, but did not influence several indicators of sleep [22]. In a further investigation of 15 patients with PD and disruptive nocturnal symptoms, sustained-release levodopa improved night-time akinesia and total time awake [23].

The usability of dopamine agonists was first investigated with the long-acting peroral dopamine agonist cabergoline, which was compared with levodopa as a medication for patients to take before sleep [24]. The results suggested that the long-acting effect of cabergoline was more beneficial to the short-acting levodopa. A further study has investigated the peroral dopamine agonist pramipexole and the transdermal dopamine agonist rotigotine in advanced stage PD [25]. Both pramipexole tablets and rotigotine patches resulted in overall improvements in the PD sleep scale: compared with placebo there was improvement in sleep akinesia and comparable results were reported with slow-release ropinirole [26]. The quality standards subcommittee of the AAN concluded that there is evidence that levodopa improves the night-time motor symptoms that can cause insomnia, but that there is insufficient evidence that levodopa causes an objective improvement in sleep quality [18]. The committee further concluded that melatonin improves the patient's feeling of sleep quality, but it is unclear if it objectively improves sleep [18].

The most compelling level 1 evidence has recently been published in the form an international randomised placebo controlled trail of rotigotine transdermal patch compared to placebo in the RECOVER study, which used the PDSS-2 and UPDRS III (early morning motor function) as co-primary outcome measures along with the NMSS as a secondary outcome measure [27]. There was a significant improvement in PDSS-2 scores which was clinically meaningful and was also reflected in a significant improvement in the sleep domain of the NMSS.These results, together with an improvement in motor state, resulted in a highly significant improvement in the HRQoL of patients. Patients with significant night-time problems, such as akinesia, early morning off and pain therefore could be reasonably be given a treatment option of the rotigotine patch [27]. Post-hoc analysis of data from two pivotal ropinirole prolonged-release studies also suggest a beneficial effect on PDSS, although the effect attenuates at 24 weeks [28,29]. More recent long-term follow-up data suggest that the effect of the rotigotine patch on sleep and motor functions is maintained at 12 months [29].

The significant improvements in patients with Parkinson's on the rotigotine transdermal patch treatment in aspects of their sleep (early morning function as well as no worsening in daytime sleepiness), pain, and mood, as reported in the RECOVER study, translates overall to a significant and robust improvement in their HRQoL [30].

In a practical clinical setting it is advisable to make a precise analysis of the possible reasons behind the patient's insomnia and to design the treatment accordingly [31]. If the reason seems to be night-time PD symptoms, levodopa or dopamine agonist medicine doses in the late evening, preferably long acting, are advisable. In case the insomnia could be a side effect of parkinsonian drugs, it might be advisable to stop the suspected drug, which can be selegiline, dopamine agonists or levodopa. In cases where depression could be a causative factor, a trial with mirtazapine or mianserine could prove effective. In patients in whom nightmares are connected with the insomnia, reduction of evening PD medication, as well as use of atypical neuroleptic drugs (quetiapine, clozapine), can be indicated.

Excessive daytime somnolence

Excessive daytime somnolence, defined as a debilitating trend to drift off to sleep, or rapid-onset sleep without any prior drowsiness, in appropriate circumstances, affects up to 50% of patients with PD and can occur early in the disease development, often predating diagnosis [5,32]. It can profoundly influence quality of life and is therefore important to detect [33,34]. Daytime somnolence is associated with poor concentration and memory and may lead to driving and/or occupational accidents [35].

The causes of daytime somnolence are multifactorial, and include the disease process itself, night-time sleep disruption, depression, and drug therapy with agents including antihistamines, dopaminergic therapies, anxiolytics and selective serotonin reuptake inhibitors (SSRIs). Haq et al [36] have suggested a secondary narcoleptic phenotype in PD connected to degeneration of hypocretin-containing neurons in the hypothalamus. Saper et al [35] propose that a 'flip-flop' switch is responsible for the sleep–wake cycle. Dopaminergic dysfunction and neural degeneration have been suggested to destabilize the switch and its regulators, promoting rapid transitions to sleep. After reports of road traffic accidents caused by sudden irresistible onset of sleep in PD patients, there was considerable interest concerning the role of dopaminergic drugs with regard to sedation and sudden onset of sleep. The results of this research indicate that not only dopamine agonists but also levodopa could be involved [37–39].

In practical clinical work, it is important to realize that excessive daytime somnolence and sudden onset of sleep can increase the risk of serious injury, particularly if the patient drives a vehicle or could be injured at work. A total of 11% of PD patients were implicated in the causation of at least one road traffic accident in the preceding 5 years, and 1–4% of patients report sudden-onset sleep while driving [40]. The level of daytime sleepiness must be regularly checked in patients with PD, especially when dopaminergic treatment is changed [40] and those at risk must not drive vehicles or operate machinery. Assessment can be made using various scales including the ESS and PDSS.

To improve these symptoms, exclusion/substitution of the suspected drugs, first-line dopamine agonists, can be tried. Treating patients with stimulants such as modafinil is only partially efficacious, whereas trials of anti-H_3-receptor drugs and sodium oxybate seem more promising [40]. Modafinil improves the patient's feeling of 'awakeness', but fails to induce an objective improvement of the tiredness [18].

Rapid eye movement sleep behavior disorder

RBD is typically characterized by vivid and frightening dreams associated with simple and complex movements during REM sleep (when the muscles are normally atonic), with the patients seeming to act out their dreams [12,41]. Bed partners report on vocalizations as well as abnormal, partly violent movements. The disorder is very debilitating for the patient and the patient's bed partner; injuries sustained have been reported to include lacerations, fracture, ecchymosis and dislocations. REM sleep without atonia (RWA) shows an abnormal occurrence of muscle activation during REM sleep but no manifesting behaviors. Definite diagnosis of RBD should be made via single-night PSG testing because clinical criteria alone have been shown to be only 33% sensitive for diagnosis [42].

RBD is thought to precede the onset of motor symptoms in over 40% of PD patients [43,44] and a latency of 12.7 years has been reported [45–47]. It has been suggested that RBD could be used, together with other early symptoms (such as olfactory disturbance, depression and constipation) and transcranial ultrasonography and FP-CIT ([^{123}I]2β-carbomethoxy-3β-(4-iodophenyl)-N-(3-fluoropropyl) nortropane) imaging, to develop premotor symptom testing for PD [48–50]. Tonic REM sleep atonia may be more predictive of parkinsonism than phasic REM sleep atonia [51].

In patients with isolated RBD, imaging studies have indicated a significant reduction in striatal dopaminergic uptake in a proportion of the patients [48]. However, the pathological basis of RBD is still unclear. A hypothesis is that RBD arises because of degeneration of lower brainstem nuclei, consistent with Braak stages 1 and 2 [52]. Degeneration of the sublaterodorsal nucleus, with its direct and indirect projections to the spinal interneurons, has been implicated as well as involvement of the laterodorsal tegmental nucleus, perilocus ceruleus region, nucleus reticularis magnocellularis, pedunculopontine nucleus and ventrolateral reticulospinal tracts [12].

There are no controlled trials for treatment of RBD, but clinical experience and open studies indicate that night-time dosing with levodopa and use of clonazepam or pramipexole may reduce involuntary nocturnal movements during sleep [53]; alternative medications for RBD might be mirtazapine and mianserine. The quality standards subcommittee of the AAN concludes that clonazepam and melatonin are often used for this indication, but that evidence for the effect of these drugs is insufficient [18].

Sleep-disordered breathing

There are limited studies reporting the frequency of sleep-disordered breathing in PD, and the figures quoted are variable, ranging from 2.5% to 66%. Obstructive sleep apnea is probably the dominant type of sleep-disordered breathing, but the frequency and clinical relevance of this problem are still being debated [54,55] and PD patients can have these problems without any increase in body mass index. Snoring, one of the symptoms of sleep apnea, has been shown to predict the occurrence of daytime somnolence. The diagnostic procedure includes sleep laboratory examination and treatment, including continuous positive airway pressure treatment, should be decided on an individual basis, according to normal routines for these symptoms. Sleep-disordered breathing might coexist with RBD, so caution should be taken when treating RBD with clonazepam, which can have a detrimental effect on sleep-disordered breathing.

References

1   Lees AJ, Blackburn NA, Campbell VL. The nighttime problems of Parkinson's disease. *Clin Neuropharmacol* 1988;11:512-519.

2   Chaudhuri KR. Nocturnal symptom complex in PD and its management. *Neurology* 2003;61:S17-S23.

3   Garcia-Borreguero D, Larosa O, Bravo M. Parkinson's disease and sleep. *Sleep Med Rev* 2003a;7:115-129.

4   Lai YY, Siegel JM. Muscle tone suppression and stepping produced by stimulation of midbrain and rostral pontine reticular formation. *J Neurol* 1990;10:2727-2734.

5   Rye DB, Jankovic J. Emerging views of dopamine in modulating sleep/wake state from an unlikely source: PD. *Neurology* 2002;58:341-346.

6   Arnulf I, Konofal E, Merino-Andreu M, et al. Parkinson's disease and sleepiness – an integral part of PD. *Neurology* 2002;58:1019-1024.

7   Mehta SH, Morgan JC, Sethi KD. Sleep disorders associated with Parkinson's disease: role of dopamine, epidemiology, and clinical scales of assessment. *CNS Spectr* 200813(Suppl 4):6-11.

8   Kunz D, Mahlberg R. A two-part, double-blind, placebo-controlled trial of exogenous melatonin in REM sleep behavior disorder. *J Sleep Res* 2010; 19:591-596.

9   Schapira AH. Restless legs syndrome: an update on treatment options. *Drugs* 2004;64:149-158.

10 Muzerengi S, Lewis H, Chaudhuri KR. Restless legs syndrome: a review of diagnosis and management. Int *J Sleep Disord* 2006;1:34-46.

11 Peralta CM, Frauscher B, Seppi K, et al. Restless legs syndrome in Parkinson's disease. *Mov Disord* 2009;24:2076-2080.

12 Mitra T, Chaudhuri K. Sleep dysfunction and role of dysautonomia in Parkinson's disease. *Parkinsonism Relat Disord* 2009;15:S93-S95.

13 Möller JC, Unger M, Stiasny-Kolster K, Oertel WH. Restless legs syndrome (RLS) and Parkinson's disease (PD)-related disorders or different entities? *J Neurol Sci* 2010;289:135-137.

14 Ondo WG, Vuong KD, Jankovic J. Exploring the relationship between Parkinsons'disease and restless legs syndrome. *Arch Neurol* 2002;59:421-424.

15 Garcia-Borreguero D, Odin P, Serrano C. Restless legs syndrome and Parkinson: A review of the evidence for a possible association. *Neurology* 2003b;61:49-55.

16 Reuter I, Ellis CM, Chaudhuri KR. Nocturnal subcutaneous apomorphine infusion in Parkinson's disease and restless legs syndrome. *Acta Neurol Scand* 1999;100:163-167.

17 Högl B, Rotdach A, Wetter TC, Trenkwalder C. The effect of cabergoline on sleep, periodic leg movements in sleep and early morning motor function in patients with Parkinson's disease. *Neuropsychopharmacology* 2003;28:1866-1870.

18 Zesiewicz TA, Sullivan KL, Arnulf I; for Quality Standards Subcommittee of the American Academy of Neurology Practice. Parameter: treatment of nonmotor symptoms of Parkinson disease: report of the Quality Standards Subcommittee of the American Academy of Neurology. *Neurology* 2010;74:924-931.

19 Chaudhuri K, Schapira A. Non-motor symptoms of Parkinson's disease: dopaminergic pathophysiology and treatment. *Lancet Neurol* 2009;8:464-474.

20 Dhawan V, Healy DG, Pal S, Chaudhuri KR. Sleep-related problems in Parkinson's disease. *Age Aging* 2006;35:220-228.

21 Leeman AL, O'Neill CJ, Nicholson PW, et al. Parkinson's disease in the elderly: response to and optimal spacing of night-time dosing with levodopa. *Br J Clin Pharmacol* 1987;24:637-643.

22 Stocchi F, Barbato L, Nordera G, et al. Sleep disorders in Parkinson's disease. *J Neurol* 1998;245:S15-S18.

23 Van der Kerchowe M, Jacquy J, Gonce M, et al. Sustained-release levodopa in parkinsonian patients with nocturnal disabilities. *Acta Neurol Belg* 1993;93:32-39.

24 Chaudhuri KR, Bhattacharya K, Agapito C, et al. The use of cabergoline in nocturnal parkinsonian disabilities causing sleep disruption: a parallel study with controlled-release levodopa. *Eur J Neurol* 1999;6:S11-S15.

25 Poewe W, Rascol O, Quinn N, et al; on behalf of the Sp515 investigators. Efficacy of pramipexole and transdermal rotigotine in advanced Parkinson's disease: a double blind, double dummy randomized controlled trial. *Lancet Neurol* 2007;6:513-520.

26 Pahwa R, Stady MA, Factor SA, et al; on behalf of the EASE-PD adjunct study investigators. Ropinirole 24 hours prolonged release randomized controlled study in advanced Parkinson's disease. *Neurology* 2007;68:1108-1115.

27 Trenkwalder C, Kies B, Rudsinska M, et al; and the RECOVER study group. Rotigotine effects on early morning motor function and sleep in Parkinson's disease: A double-blind, randomised, placebo-controlled study (RECOVER). *Mov Disord* 2011;26:90-99.

28 Chaudhuri KR, Martinez-Martin P, Rolfe KA, et al. Improvements in nocturnal symptoms with ropinirole prolonged release in patients with advanced Parkinson's disease. *Eur J Neurol* 2011. E-Pub. doi: 10.1111/j.1468-1331.2011.03442.x

29 Trenkwalder C, Zucconi M, Tolosa E, et al. Effects of transdermal rotigotine on sleep and nocturnal symptoms over a 1-year period in Parkinson's disease: an open-label extension of the RECOVER study. In: Proceedings from the World Association of Sleep Medicine and Canadian Sleep Society Congress; September 10-15, 2011; Quebec City, Canada. Abstract M-E-053.

30 Ghys L, Surmann E, Whitesides J, Boroojerdi B. Effect of rotigotine on sleep and quality of life in Parkinson's disease patients: post hoc analysis of RECOVER patients who were symptomatic at baseline. *Expert Opin Pharmacother* 2011;12:1985-1998.

31 Korczyn AD. Management of sleep problems in Parkinson's disease. *J Neurol Sci* 2006;248:163-166.

32 Abbott RD, Ross GW, White LR, et al. Excessive daytime sleepiness and the risk of Parkinson's disease. *Mov Disord* 2005;20:S101.

33 Schapira AH. Excessive daytime sleepiness in Parkinson's disease. *Neurology* 2004;63:S24-S27.

34 Macmahon D. Why excessive daytime sleepiness is an important issue in Parkinson's disease. *Adv Clin Neurol Rehab* 2005;5:46-49.

35 Saper C, Chou TC, Scammell TE. The sleep switch: Hypothalamic control of sleep and wakefulness. *Trends Neurosci* 2001;24:726-731.

36 Haq I, Naidu Y, Reddy P, Chaudhuri KR. Narcolepsy in Parkinson's disease. *Exp Rev Neurother* 2010;10:879-884.

37 Andreu N, Chale J-J, Senard J-M, et al. L-Dopa-induced sedation: a double-blind cross-over controlled study versus trazolam and placebo in healthy volunteers. *Clin Neuropharmacol* 1999;22:15-23.

38 Frucht S, Rogers JD, Greene PE, et al. Falling asleep at the wheel: motor vehicle mishaps in persons taking pramipexole and ropinirole. *Neurology* 1999;52:1908-1910.

39 Ferreira JJ, Galitzky M, Montastruc JL, Rascol O. Sleep attacks in Parkinson's disease. *Lancet* 2000;355:1333-1334.

40 Arnulf I, Leu-Semenescu S. Sleepiness in Parkinson's disease. *Parkinsonism Relat Disord* 2009;15(suppl 3):S101-S104.

41 Boeve BF, Silber MH, Saper B, et al. Pathophysiology of REM sleep behavior disorder and relevance to neurodegenerative disease. *Brain* 2007;130:2770-2788.

42 Comella C. Sleep disorders in Parkinson's disease: an overview. *Mov Disord* 2007;22:S367-S373.

43 Schenck CH, Bundle SR, Mahowald MW. Delayed emergence of a parkinsonian disorder in 38% of 29 older men initially diagnosed with idiopathic rapid eye movement sleep behavior disorder. *Neurology* 1996;46:388-393.

44 Chaudhuri KR, Healy DG, Schapira AH. Non-motor symptoms of Parkinson's disease: Diagnosis and management. *Lancet Neurol* 2006;5:235-245.

45 Tan A, Salgado M, Fahn S. Rapid eye movement sleep behavior disorder preceding Parkinson's disease with therapeutic response to levodopa. *Mov Disord* 1996;11:214-216.

46 Schenck CH, Mahowald ME. REM-sleep behavior disorder: clinical, developmental and neuroscience perspectives 16 years after its formal identification in SLEEP. *Sleep* 2002;25:120-138.

47 Iranzo A, Molinuevo JL, Santamaria J, et al. Rapid-eye movement sleep behavior disorder as an early marker for neurodegenerative disorder: a descriptive study. *Lancet Neurol* 2006;5:572-577.

48 Eisensehr I, Linke R, Noachtar S, et al. Reduced striatal dopamine transporters in idiopathic rapid eye movement sleep behavior disorder: Comparison with Parkinson's disease and controls. *Brain* 2000;123:1155-1160.

49 Stiasny-Kolster K, Doerr Y, Moller JC, et al. Combination of idiopathic REM sleep behavior disorder and olfactory dysfunction as possible indicator for alpha-synucleinopathy demonstrated by dopamine transporter FP-CIT-SPECT. *Brain* 2005;128:126-137.

50 Unger MM, Moeller JC, Stiasny-Kolster K, et al. Assessment of idiopathic rapid-eye-movement sleep behavior disorder by transcranial sonography, olfactory function test, and FP-CIT-SPECT. *Mov Disord* 2008;23:596-599.

51 Postuma RB, Gagnon JF, Rompre S, Montplaisir JY. Severity of REM atonia loss in idiopathic REM sleep behavior disorder predicts Parkinson disease. *Neurology* 2010;74:239-244.

52 Wolters E, Braak J. Parkinson's disease: Premotor clinico-pathological correlations. *J Neurol Transm* 2006;79:309-319.

53 Olson EJ, Boeve BF, Silber MH. Rapid eye movement sleep behavior disorder: demographic, clinical and laboratory findings in 93 cases. *Brain* 2000;123:331-339.

54 Cochen De Cock V, Abouda M, Leu S, et al. Is obstructive sleep apnea a problem in Parkinson's disease? *Sleep Med* 2010;11:247-252.

55 Högl B. Sleep apnea in Parkinson's disease: when is it significant? *Sleep Med* 2010;11:233-235.

Chapter 7

Bladder dysfunction

Angelo Antonini

Bladder dysfunction is a common complaint in elderly people with multifactorial origin. It is also frequent in Parkinson's disease (PD) [1,2],
and is an important cause of impairment of health-related quality of life
(HRQoL) leading to considerable disability and handicap. Urinary dysfunction in PD manifests primarily with symptoms of overactive bladder
(OAB) – ie increased frequency and urgency of micturition or urge incontinence – and correlates well with urodynamic findings of involuntary
detrusor contractions at early stages of bladder filling (detrusor hyperflexia) [3,4]. Bladder dysfunctions occur also in atypical parkinsonism
and particularly as an early manifestation of multiple system atrophy
(MSA) in which urinary retention is more common [5].

Prevalence

The first studies to look at the prevalence of lower urinary tract symptoms
(LUTs) in PD showed a high incidence of neurogenic detrusor overactivity, although there was probably an element of pre-selection in patient
groups [6]. Early studies suggest that urinary dysfunction affects between
37% and 70% of PD patients [7,8]. A recent international survey used the
Non-Motor Symptom Questionnaire (NMSQuest – self-completed non-
motor questionnaire) to examine non-motor symptoms (NMSs) of PD
in 545 patients with a mean Hoehn and Yahr (H&Y) stage of 2.5 [9,10].

K. R. Chaudhuri et al., *Handbook of Non-Motor Symptoms
in Parkinson's Disease*, DOI: 10.1007/978-1-908517-60-9_7,
© Springer Healthcare, a part of Springer Science+Business Media 2011

This survey found that 56% answered positively to the question 'Have you experienced a sense of urgency to pass urine which makes you rush to the toilet?', but the question 'Have you experienced getting up early at night to pass urine?' got the highest response at 62%. It also emerged that 'urinary' had the highest percentage of positive answers of all nine symptom domains [10].

A similar global prevalence study of NMSs has also been recently reported. The PRIAMO (Parkinson's and Non Motor Symptoms) Study analyzed NMSs and their relationship with QoL in over 1000 Italian PD patients. The urinary dysfunction was reported in 57.3%, ranging from 37.7% in early PD (H&Y stage 1) to 89.8% (H&Y stage 4–5) [11].

The underlying pathophysiology of symptoms

Dopaminergic mechanisms are thought to play an important role in normal micturition control. Dopaminergic neurons have both inhibitory and stimulatory effects on micturition acting via D_1 and D_2-receptors, respectively. Such neurons are of particular abundance in the substantia nigra pars compacta (SNC) and the ventral tegmental area (VTA) of the midbrain. Dysfunction of these mechanisms may lead to detrusor overactivity (DO). The most widely accepted theory is that basal ganglia inhibit the micturition reflex in the normal situation via D_1-receptors, and cell depletion in SNC in idiopathic PD results in loss of D_1-receptor-mediated inhibition and consequently DO [12,13].

Studies suggest that severity of urinary dysfunction may also correlate with the relative degeneration of the caudate nucleus, which receives dopamine-rich innervations from the SNC and VTA [14].

It has been shown that deep brain stimulation at the subthalamic nucleus leads to improved sensory motor integration, and there also is evidence that higher-order processing of afferent activity is improved in patients with PD whose bladder symptoms are ameliorated by medication [15].

Thus, the notion that DO is the main underlying problem resulting from the loss of dopamine-mediated inhibition may be an oversimplification, and it is likely that this symptomatology arises from a combination of factors.

Clinical manifestations

LUTSs are classified as irritative and obstructive symptoms. In the irritative group there is frequency, urgency and nocturia, which are caused by hyperactivity of the bladder due to detrusor hyperflexia. Detrusor hyperflexia refers to a hyperactive bladder, whereas incomplete emptying, intermittent weak urinary stream and hesitation are obstructive symptoms (Figure 7.1).

It is widely accepted that the complaint of urinary urgency reflects underlying DO, which has repeatedly been shown to be the common urodynamic abnormality in patients with PD and symptoms of an OAB. However, symptoms of voiding difficulty are also known to occur. The background behind incomplete voiding is less clear, although authors have suggested that it might be a consequence of insufficient bladder contractility [16].

The most prevalent urinary symptom in idiopathic DP is 'nocturia' (up to 86%), followed by 'urgency' (33–71%) and 'frequency' (16–68%) [17,18]. These may lead to urinary incontinence, which would be in part functional if immobility or poor manual dexterity did not complicate the situation. The reason for this complaint has not been properly elucidated, and possible explanations lie with an increased urine output at night, reduced bladder capacity or impairment of sleep. Although DO, which commonly affects patients with PD would be expected to result in a reduced bladder capacity and thus increased frequency, the nocturia

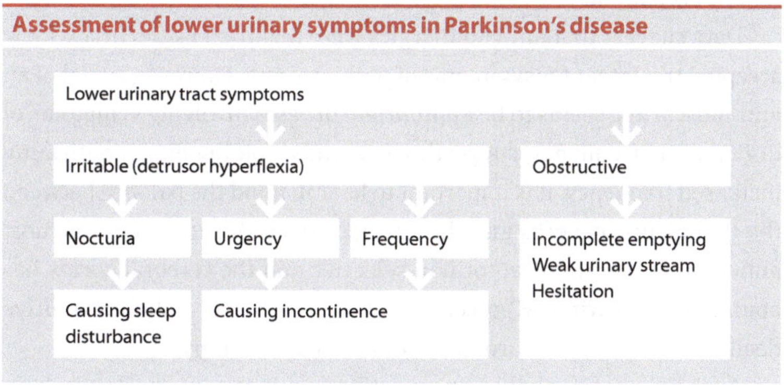

Assessment of lower urinary symptoms in Parkinson's disease

Lower urinary tract symptoms

Irritable (detrusor hyperflexia) | Obstructive

Nocturia | Urgency | Frequency | Incomplete emptying / Weak urinary stream / Hesitation

Causing sleep disturbance | Causing incontinence

Figure 7.1 Assessment of lower urinary symptoms in Parkinson's disease.

appears to be disproportionate compared with the daytime frequency, suggesting additional mechanisms.

Treatment and management

The history provided by the patient or caregiver plays a crucial role in the recognition of urinary dysfunction in PD. In addition, health professionals may find it convenient to ask patients and their caregivers to maintain a 3-day 24-hour bladder dairy. This method may be useful in getting a detailed record of the time and volume of each void along with the sensation preceding the void (urgency).

The only agreed finding from various studies is that voiding difficulty is less when individuals are 'on' (with their symptoms well-controlled) [19]. Nevertheless findings in respect to the acute effect of levodopa are contradictory and both aggravation and alleviation of bladder symptoms are reported [20–22]. This may be explained by the observation that, in patients with advanced disease and motor fluctuations, levodopa worsened DO during bladder filling, but facilitated voiding by exerting a relatively greater effect on detrusor contractility compared with external sphincter closure [16].

Moreover, the dopamine agonist apomorphine has been shown to improve voiding efficiency by increasing urine flow and reducing post-void residual urine volume (PVR), although its effect on detrusor muscle may vary. Figure 7.2 gives a management strategy for urinary dysfunction in PD patients.

Data suggest that anticholinergics were regarded as the first widely accepted treatment for symptoms of parkinsonism. However, a trial of an anti-muscarinic seems to be appropriate in cases involving symptoms of urgency and frequency, suggesting DO, and a voiding diary confirming increased frequency. It is important to bear in mind the balance between the therapeutic benefits and the adverse effects of such drugs. As most anticholinergics are receptor non-selective and the cerebral cortex has abundant muscarinic M_1-receptors, there is a concern about cognitive decline in response to chronic anti-muscarinic therapy.

Anticholinergics should be prescribed with caution, particularly in patients presenting with hallucinations or cognitive decline (or demen-

Management strategy for urinary dysfunction in Parkinson's disease
Bladder diary (24-h for 3 days)
Wearing off-related detrusor overactivity
Continuous drug delivery (may facilitate voiding)
CR levodopa
Rotigotine patch/ER pramipexole and ER ropinirole
Apomorphine infusion
Levodopa intrajejunal infusion
Urgency and frequency
Anticholinergic
Oxybutynin
Solifenacin (fewer side effects)
General
Urinary review
Self-catherization

Figure 7.2 Management strategy for urinary dysfunction in Parkinson's disease.
CR, controlled release; ER, extended release.

tia); for example, trihexyphenidyl (for PD) and oxybutynin (for OAB) have been shown to have central side effects. Blocking of M_3-receptors in the salivary glands can lead to dry mouth, whereas constipation may develop due to blocking of both M_2- and M_3-receptors in bowel. However, despite these restrictions, anticholinergic therapy, when appropriately monitored, remains a valid treatment option for urinary dysfunction in PD.

Finally, patients should be referred to a urologist for further investigation, if persisting urinary symptoms are related to possible bladder outlet obstruction.

References

1 Sakakibara R, Hattori T, Uchiyama T, Yamanishi T. Videourodynamic and sphincter motor unit potential analyses in Parkinson's disease and multiple system atrophy. *J Neurol Neurosurg Psychiatry* 2001;71:600-606.

2 Hely MA, Morris JG, Reid WG, Trafficante R. Sydney multicenter study of Parkinson's disease: non-L-dopa-responsive problems dominate at 15 years. *Mov Disord* 2005;20:190-199.

3 Singer C. Urinary dysfunction in Parkinson's disease. *Clin Neurosci* 1998;5:78-86.

4 Defreitas GA, Lemack GE, Zimmern PE, Dewey RB, Roehrborn CG, O'Suilleabhain PE. Distinguishing neurogenic from non-neurogenic detrusor overactivity: a urodynamic assessment of lower urinary tract symptoms in patients with and without Parkinson's disease. *Urology* 2003;62:651-655.

5   Winge K, Fowler CJ. Scientific evidence and expert clinical opinion for the investigation and management of incontinence and sexual dysfunction. In: Findley L, Hurwitz B, Miles A (eds), *The Effective Management of Parkinson's Disease*. London: Aesculapius Medical Press, 2004: 149-156.

6   Araki I, Kuno S. Assessment of voiding dysfunction in Parkinson's disease by the international prostate symptom score. *J Neurol Neurosurg Psychiatry* 2000;68:429-433.

7   Andersen JT, Bradley WE. Cystometric, sphincter and electromyelographic abnormalities in Parkinson's disease. *J Urol* 1976;116:75-78.

8   Berger Y, Blaivas JG, DeLaRocha ER, Salinas JM. Urodynamic findings in Parkinson's disease. *J Urol* 1987;138:836-838.

9   Chaudhuri KR, Martinez-Martin P, Schapira AH, et al. International multicenter pilot study of the first comprehensive self-completed nonmotor symptoms questionnaire for Parkinson's disease: the NMSQuest study. *Mov Disord* 2006;21:916-923.

10 Martinez-Martin P, Schapira AH, Stocchi F, et al. Prevalence of nonmotor symptoms in Parkinson's disease in an international setting; Study using nonmotor symptoms questionnaire in 545 patients. *Mov Disord* 2007;22:1623-1629.

11 Barone P, Antonini A, Colosimo C, et al;.for the PRIAMO Study. A multicenter assessment of non-motor symptoms and their impact on quality of life in Parkinson's disease. *Mov Disord* 2009;24:1641-1649.

12 Yoshimura N, Mizuta E, Kuno S, Yoshida O. The mechanism for inducing detrusor hyperreflexia in the primate model of parkinsonism. *Neurourol Urodyn* 1990;9:371.

13 Seki S, Igawa Y, Kaidoh K, et al. Role of dopamine D1 and D1 receptors in the micturition reflex in conscious rats. *Neurourol Urodyn* 2001;20:105-113.

14 Winge K, Friberg L, Werdelin L, Nielson K, Stimpel H. Relationship between nigrostriatal dopaminergic degeneration, urinary symptoms, and bladder control in Parkinson's disease. *Eur J Neurol* 2005;12:842-850.

15 Winge K, Werdelin LM, Nielsen KK, Stimpel H. Effects of dopaminergic treatment on bladder function in Parkinson's disease. *Neurourol Urodyn* 2004;23:689-696.

16 Uchiyama T, Sakakibara R, Hattori T, Yamanishi T. Short-term effect of a single levodopa dose on micturition disturbance in Parkinson's disease patients with the wearing-off phenomenon. *Mov Disord* 2003;18:573-578.

17 Campos-Sousa R, Quagliato E, Da Silva B, de Carvalho R Jr, Ribiero S, de Carvalho D. Urinary symptoms in Parkinson's disease: prevalence and associated factors. *Arquivos de Neuro-Psiquiatria* 2003;61:67-71.

18 Winge K, Skau A, Stimpel H, Nielson K, Werdelin L. Prevalence of bladder dysfunction in Parkinson's disease. *Neurourol Urodyn* 2006;25:116-122.

19 Antonini A, Tolosa E, Mizuno Y, Yamamoto M, Poewe WA. Reasssessment of risks and benefits of dopamine agonists in Parkinson's disease. *Lancet Neurol* 2009;8:929-937.

20 Fitzmaurice H, Fowler CJ, Rickards D. Micturition disturbance in Parkinson's disease. *Br J Urol* 1985;57:652-656.

21 Christmas T, Chapple C, Lees A, Frankel J, Stern G, Milroy E. Role of subcutaneous apomorphine in parkinsonian voiding dysfunction. *Lancet* 1988;ii:1451-1453.

22 Aranda B, Cramer P. Effects of apomorphine and L-dopa on the parkinsonian bladder. *Neurourol Urodyn* 1993;12:203-209.

Chapter 8

Sensory symptoms

K Ray Chaudhuri

Sensory disturbances are among the most common non-motor symptoms (NMSs), experienced by between 30% and 95% of patients with Parkinson's disease (PD) [1]. Nevertheless, sensory NMSs remain under-reported, under-recognized and poorly understood. Similarly, controversy, misconceptions and uncertainty surround fatigue and weight change, which are also common NMSs among PD patients.

Health-care professionals can assess many sensory dysfunctions using NMSQuest (see Chapter 4).

Olfactory dysfunction

Since the first description of PD-related hyposmia in 1975 [2], compelling evidence emerged suggesting that most idiopathic PD patients show olfactory dysfunction [3]. Indeed, all PD subtypes appear to induce hyposmia [4], which arises from both orthonasal and retronasal olfactory dysfunction.

In many PD patients, olfactory dysfunction precedes motor symptoms by several years. Indeed, more than 95% of PD patients show significant hyposmia on presentation [5]. According to the six-stage pathological process proposed by Braak and colleagues (see Figure 1.2) [6], Lewy bodies initially form in the olfactory bulb and anterior olfactory nucleus, producing olfactory dysfunction. During the second stage, Lewy bodies

K. R. Chaudhuri et al., *Handbook of Non-Motor Symptoms in Parkinson's Disease*, DOI: 10.1007/978-1-908517-60-9_8,
© Springer Healthcare, a part of Springer Science+Business Media 2011

form in the lower brain-stem nuclei, which probably also contributes to a range of NMSs, including olfaction, sleep disturbances, depression and cognition, pain, constipation, and dysfunctional central autonomic vagal control. Several of these NMSs are possible premotor features of PD [7].

Numerous studies suggest that olfactory dysfunction is common among people with PD. In a prospective study of 45 PD patients, patients correctly identified 56% and 60% of orthonasal and retronasal stimuli, respectively [3]. Haehner et al [5], who evaluated 400 PD patients using a psychophysical olfactory test, found that 45% were functionally anosmic, 51.7% were hyposmic and 3.3% were normosmic. Overall, 96.7% and 74.5% of PD patients presented with significant olfactory loss compared with population- and age-matched norms, respectively.

As mentioned above, olfactory dysfunction probably follows aggregation of Lewy bodies and α-synuclein in the olfactory bulb [4]. However, the severity of olfactory impairment appears to be independent of PD duration, stage or treatment [3]. Against this background, physicians should assess olfactory function during the differential diagnosis of suspected PD [3]. Indeed, Hawkes [8] argues that normal olfactory function should prompt a reconsideration of the differential diagnosis of idiopathic PD; for example, hyposmia does not occur in progressive supranuclear palsy or corticobasal degeneration, and is less common in multiple system atrophy compared with PD [4]. Furthermore, as hyposmia may contribute to inadequate nutrition, clinicians should regularly assess olfactory function.

Changes in visual function

PD is associated with several ocular disturbances (Figure 8.1), including blurred vision, dry eyes, difficulty reading, diplopia, fatigue of eye movements, impaired color discrimination and contrast deficits. Moreover, between 25% and 40% of PD patients experience visual hallucinations [10]. Impaired color discrimination and contrast deficits, in particular, often emerge before motor symptoms [11], and seem to be associated with an increased risk of visual hallucinations. Not surprisingly, PD-associated visual disturbances can markedly impair activities of daily living, including ambulation, negotiating stairs and driving [12];

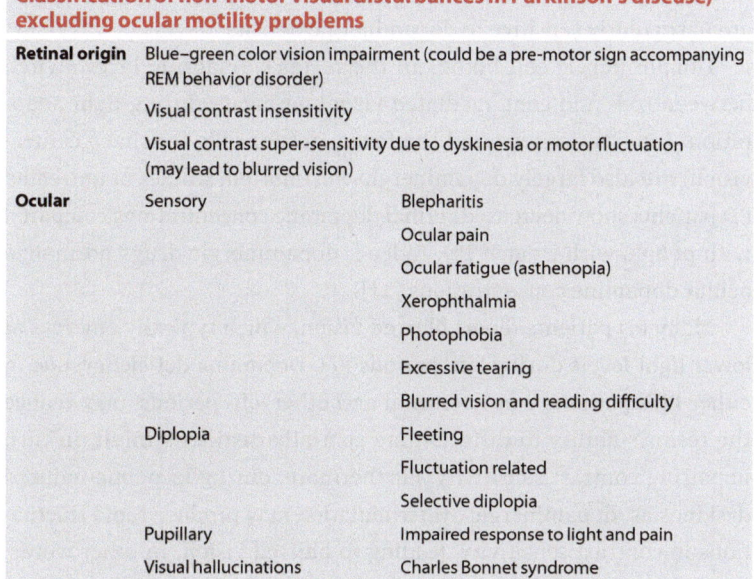

Figure 8.1 Classification of non-motor visual disturbances in Parkinson's disease, excluding ocular motility problems. REM, rapid eye movement. Data from Hawkes [9].

for example, PD patients enduring visuospatial dysfunction may bump into doorways and be at increased risk of falls.

Reduced color discrimination is one of the visual hallmarks of PD; for example, Büttner and colleagues [11] performed the Farnsworth–Munsell 100-hue color discrimination test in 16 new PD patients and 16 age-matched controls. PD patients made more discriminatory errors than controls (means of 64.6 and 16.0, respectively). The same group compared chromatic fusion time (CFT), which indicates perceptual acuity for monochromatic contours, in 28 previously untreated PD patients and 28 age- and sex-matched controls. PD patients showed shortened CFT, especially for light-blue and dark-green contours. The extent of the abnormal chromatic perception correlated with PD severity [13]. As this study found, PD patients seem to experience particular problems discriminating the tritan (blue–green) axis. This impairment probably reflects the relatively low number of blue–green cones in the retina and a relative lack of inhibition of the surrounding neurons (surround inhibition accentuates excited retinal regions). As a result, blue–green cones are particularly sensitive to dopaminergic deficits.

Dopaminergic cell bodies in the retina's amacrine layer switch between rod- and cone-mediated visual pathways during light adaptation. Innervations around the fovea (responsible for sharp central vision) are also largely dopaminergic. Postmortem studies of untreated PD patients show decreased retinal dopamine concentrations compared with people with treated PD. Indeed, dopaminergic drugs normalize ocular dopamine concentrations [11].

Many PD patients report blurred vision, which typically emerges at lower light levels during 'off' periods [7]. Dopamine deficiency, due to either PD's pathology or nocturnal and other 'off' periods, may reduce the retina's ability to differentiate spatially distinct stimuli, in turn impairing contrast sensitivity. Furthermore, during levodopa-induced dyskinesias, dopaminergic overstimulation may produce rapid fluctuations in contrast sensitivity, leading to blurred vision. In other words, retinal dopaminergic deficiency probably accounts for several visual NMSs among PD patients, including decreased color discrimination and visuospatial deficits. Obviously, retinal dopaminergic deficiency does not underlie extraretinal visual NMSs, such as visual hallucinations, abnormal ocular or eyelid movements (including diplopia) and ocular discomfort or pain (see Chapter 11).

Mild ocular disturbances may not require treatment or referral to an ophthalmologist. However, health-care professionals should offer patients advice about driving, consider asking an occupational therapist to assess the home environment, and exclude other disorders. Indeed, ocular examination can aid the differential diagnosis of PD; for example, a pupil diameter after dark adaptation of 3.99 mm differentiated progressive supranuclear palsy from PD and other extrapyramidal disorders with a specificity and sensitivity of 86.4% and 70.8%, respectively [14]. Artificial tears may alleviate xerophthalmia and blepharitis, whereas dopaminergic drugs with sustained duration of effect may improve 'off' period oculomotor symptoms.

References

1   Ansari KA, Johnson A. Olfactory function in patients with Parkinson's disease. *J Chron Dis* 1975;28:493-497.

2   Braak H, Del Tredici K, Rüb U, et al. Staging of brain pathology related to sporadic Parkinson's disease. *Neurobio Aging* 2003;24:197-210.

3   Büttner T, Kuhn W, Muller T, et al. Distorted color discrimination in 'de novo' parkinsonian patients. *Neurology* 1995;45:386-387.

4   Büttner T, Kuhn W, Przuntek H. Alterations in chromatic contour perception in de novo parkinsonian patients. *Eur Neurol* 1995;35:226-229.

5   Bye L, Vamadevan P, Chaudhuri KR. Ophthalmological aspects of Parkinson's disease. In: Chaudhuri KR, Tolosa E, Schpira A, Poewe W (eds), *Non Motor Symptoms of Parkinson's Disease*. Oxford: Oxford University Press, 2009:297-308.

6   Chaudhuri K, Schapira A. Non-motor symptoms of Parkinson's disease: dopaminergic pathophysiology and treatment. *Lancet Neurol* 2009;8:464-474.

7   Haehner A, Boesveldt S, Berendse HW, et al. Prevalence of smell loss in Parkinson's disease – a multicenter study. *Parkinsonism Relat Disord* 2009;15:490-494.

8   Haehner A, Hummel T, Reichmann H. Olfactory dysfunction as a diagnostic marker for Parkinson's disease. *Expert Rev Neurother* 2009;9:1773-1779.

9   Hawkes CH. Olfactory testing in parkinsonism. *Lancet Neurol* 2004;3:393-394.

10 Kesler A, Korczyn AD. Visual disturbances in Parkinson's disease. *Pract Neurol* 2006;6:28-33.

11 Landis BN, Cao Van H, Guinand N, et al. Retronasal olfactory function in Parkinson's disease. *Laryngoscope* 2009;119:2280-2283.

12 Zesiewicz TA, Cimino CR, Malek AR, et al. Driving safety in Parkinson's disease. *Neurology* 2002;59:1787-1788.

13 Ziemssen T, Reichmann H. Non-motor dysfunction in Parkinson's disease. *Parkinsonism Relat Disord* 2007;13:323-332.

14 Schmidt C, Herting B, Prieur S, et al. Pupil diameter in darkness differentiates progressive supranuclear palsy (PSP) from other extrapyramidal syndromes. *Mov Disord* 2007:22;2123–2126.

Chapter 9

Sexual symptoms

Angelo Antonini

Introduction

Sexual dysfunction is frequently experienced by patients with Parkinson's disease (PD) [1,2] and it is often poorly discussed or investigated in clinical patient evaluations [3,4]. Figure 9.1 lists many of the sexual problems associated with PD. The use of certain medications for PD (eg, selective serotonin reuptake inhibitors used for comorbid depression) and advanced disease stage may contribute to the development of sexual dysfunction [4,5].

Studies have indicated that the need for intimacy and sexual expression are important to the quality of life (QoL) of patients with PD. Results from a survey of 124 patients with PD found that both QoL and quality of sexual life are significantly correlated with general life satisfaction [3].

Pathophysiology

The exact pathophysiology of sexual dysfunction in PD is not fully known. However, it is hypothesized that disturbances to the meso-cortical and mesolimbic dopaminergic pathways may be involved [6]. Libido and erection are thought to be regulated by the hypothalamus, particularly the medial preoptic area (MPOA), the main integrative site for male sexual behavior [7,8]. Dopamine may help to facilitate sexual behavior, as scans of healthy volunteers during orgasm and ejaculation

K. R. Chaudhuri et al., *Handbook of Non-Motor Symptoms in Parkinson's Disease*, DOI: 10.1007/978-1-908517-60-9_9, © Springer Healthcare, a part of Springer Science+Business Media 2011

Overview of sexual problems in Parkinson's disease
Both men and women
Reduced sexual desire
Hypersexuality and increased sexual drive
Inappropriate sexual approach
Arousal problems
Orgasmic problems
Sexual dissatisfaction
Inability or limitation in intimate touching
Limited choice of sexual positions
Difficulties in sexual communication
Need for adequate planning of sexual activity (time, location, position, sexual aids)
Men
Erectile dysfunction
Premature ejaculation
Delayed ejaculation
Women
Lack of or reduced vaginal lubrication
Painful intercourse or secondary vaginismus
Difficulties reaching orgasm
Involuntary urination

Figure 9.1 Overview of sexual problems in Parkinson's disease.

showed strong activation in the dopamine-rich ventral tegmental area and mesodiencephalic junction [4,8,9].

In the paraventricular nucleus, dopamine activates oxytogenergic neurons that project to the hippocampus, medulla oblongata, and spinal cord, all of which play important roles in sexual motivation and reward [4,10].

Increasing age is the main reason for the development of sexual dysfunction in the general population [11], so this must be taken into account in patients with PD. Sexual dysfunction in PD specifically may be due to other factors besides age and loss of motor and nerve function, such as depression, the stress of having the disease, and loss of energy [12]. Partners of patients with PD, particularly female partners of male patients, also have greatly reduced sexual satisfaction. Reasons for this include not being able to share a bed with their partner due to tremors and other motor symptoms, the stress of being a caregiver, and their partners' impaired cognition and bodily functions [12,13].

Prevalence

The prevalence of general sexual dysfunction in PD ranges from 36% to 65% [5,13]. Over two-thirds of male patients have erectile dysfunction (ED) [5], while 70% of female patients have decreased libido [14]. A few studies have looked at sexual symptoms in patients with PD versus controls. Jacobs and colleagues studied 121 younger men and women with PD and 126 age- and sex-matched controls. Those with PD were more dissatisfied with their present sexual functioning and relationships and had slightly less frequent sexual intercourse [15]. Another study analyzed 84 patients with PD and 356 healthy controls, and found that the frequency of decreased libido, sexual intercourse, orgasm, erection, and ejaculation was significantly higher in patients with PD [16]. Women with PD are more likely to have anxiety or inhibition during sex, vaginal tightness, and involuntary urination, and are more prone to depression than women without PD [17].

Treatment of erectile dysfunction

Because dopamine plays a key role in male sexual arousal, dopaminergic agonists that are used to treat other PD symptoms, such as apomorphine and pergolide mesylate, may be helpful in inducing erections [2,18]. Ropinole, another dopaminergic agonist, has been shown to cause involuntary erections [18]. However, a side effect of dopamine therapy for PD is the development of impulse control disorders, including hypersexuality and other forms of sexual obsession [19,20]. Hypersexuality is controlled by reducing the dose of the dopamine agonist, switching to a more continuous dopaminergic delivery, or adding an acetylcholinesterase inhibitor, antidepressant, or antipsychotic to the treatment regimen [4,19].

The phosphodiesterase-5 inhibitor sildenafil is effective for treating ED in patients with PD [21,22]. While orthostatic hypotension is much less common in patients with PD than in those with multiple system atrophy, it is recommended that standing and lying blood pressure be measured before prescribing this agent [21]. Sildenafil also cannot be given in conjunction with nitrate therapy for cardiac disorders [2,23]. No other phosphodiesterase-5 inhibitors have been studied in the context of PD.

Treatment of general sexual dysfunction

Deep brain stimulation (DBS) in the subthalamic nucleus is often used to treat the motor symptoms of PD (eg, dyskinesia, tremor), and it may lead to improvement of sexual dissatisfaction, especially in men under 60 years of age [24]. However, there are reports of the development of transient mania with hypersexuality following DBS [25].

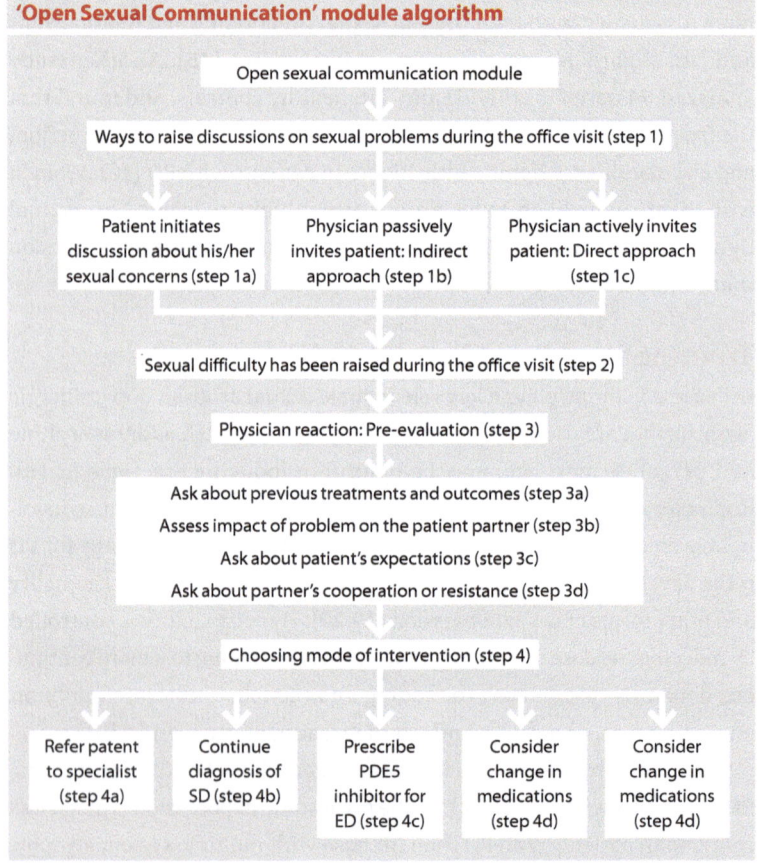

'Open Sexual Communication' module algorithm

Open sexual communication module

Ways to raise discussions on sexual problems during the office visit (step 1)

Patient initiates discussion about his/her sexual concerns (step 1a)

Physician passively invites patient: Indirect approach (step 1b)

Physician actively invites patient: Direct approach (step 1c)

Sexual difficulty has been raised during the office visit (step 2)

Physician reaction: Pre-evaluation (step 3)

Ask about previous treatments and outcomes (step 3a)
Assess impact of problem on the patient partner (step 3b)
Ask about patient's expectations (step 3c)
Ask about partner's cooperation or resistance (step 3d)

Choosing mode of intervention (step 4)

Refer patent to specialist (step 4a)

Continue diagnosis of SD (step 4b)

Prescribe PDE5 inhibitor for ED (step 4c)

Consider change in medications (step 4d)

Consider change in medications (step 4d)

Figure 9.2 'Open Sexual Communication' module algorithm. ED, erectile dysfunction; PDE5, phosphodiesterase-5; SD, sexual dysfunction. Reproduced from Bronner [27].

Therapies that are used to treat sexual dysfunction in the general population can be also be used for patients with PD. Lubrication agents and either systemic or local hormonal replacement therapy are effective in helping women with arousal problems and decreased libido. As marital problems due to sexual dysfunction are a predominant issue for both patients with PD and their partners [26], they can benefit from sex and behavioral therapy, which provides intimacy training and teaches couples how to increase sexual communication, adapt new sexual roles according to the couple's abilities, and find new solutions for physical limitation (eg, touch, arousal, orgasm).

Healthcare providers are not always sure about how to talk about sexual dysfunction issues with patients, often due to time issues and lack of training [27]. To that end, Bronner developed an 'Open Sexual Communication' module (Figure 9.2) to help providers begin conversations and give patients a secure environment where they feel comfortable discussing sexual problems. Short questionnaires may be used alone or in conjunction with the module [27], and have been proven to be helpful in prompting dialogues [28].

References

1 Sakakibara R, Shinotoh H, Uchiyama T, et al. Questionnaire-based assessment of pelvic organ dysfunction in Parkinson's disease. *Auton Neurosci* 2001; 92:76-85.

2 Papatsoris AG, Deliveliotis C, Singer C, Papapetropoulos S. Erectile dysfunction in Parkinson's disease. *Urology* 2006;67:447-451.

3 Moore O, Gurevich T, Korczyn AD, Anca M, Shabtai H, Giladi N. Quality of sexual life in Parkinson's disease. *Parkinsonism Relat Disord* 2002;8:243-246.

4 Meco G, Rubino A, Caranova N, Valente M. Sexual dysfunction in Parkinson's disease. *Parkinsonism Relat Disord* 2008;14:451-456.

5 Bronner G, Royter V, Korczyn AD, Giladi N. Sexual dysfunction in Parkinson's disease. *J Sex Marital Ther* 2004;30:95-105.

6 Celikel E, Ozel-Kizil ET, Akbostanci MC, Cevik A. Assessment of sexual dysfunction in patients with Parkinson's disease: a case–control study. *Eur J Neurol* 2008;15:1168-1172.

7 Dominguez JM, Hull EM. Dopamine, the medial preoptic area, and male sexual behavior. *Physiol Behav* 2005;86:356-368.

8 Park K, Seo JJ, Kang HK, Ryu SB, Kim HJ, Jeong GW. A new potential of blood oxygenation level dependent (BOLD) functional MRI for evaluating cerebral centers of penile erection. *Int J Impot Res* 2001;13:73-81.

9 Rees PM, Fowler CJ, Maas CP. Sexual function in men and women with neurological disorders. *Lancet* 2007;369:512-525.

10 Argiolas A, Melis MR. The role of oxytocin and the paraventricular nucleus in the sexual behavior of male mammals. *Physiol Behav* 2004;83:309-317.

11 Lindau ST, Schumm LP, Laumann EO, Levinson W, O'Muircheartaigh CA, Waite LJ. A study of sexuality and health among older adults in the United States. *N Engl J Med* 2007;357:762-774.

12 Basson R. Sexuality and Parkinson's disease. *Parkinsonism Relat Disord* 1996;2:177-185.

13 Brown RG, Jahanshahi M, Quinn N, Marsden CD. Sexual function in patients with Parkinson's disease and their partners. *J Neurol Neurosurg Psychiatry* 1990;53:480-486.

14 Pfeiffer RF. Gastrointestinal, urological, and sexual dysfunction in Parkinson's disease. *Mov Disord* 2010;25(suppl 1):S94-S97.

15 Jacobs H, Vieregge A, Vieregge P. Sexuality in young patients with Parkinson's disease: a population based comparison with healthy controls. *J Neurol Neurosurg Psychiatry* 2000;69:550-552.

16 Sakakibara R, Uchiyama T, Yamanishi T, Kishi M, et al. Genitourinary dysfunction in Parkinson's disease. *Mov Disord* 2010;25:2-12.

17 Welsh M, Hung L, Waters CH. Sexuality in women with Parkinson's disease. *Mov Disord* 1997;12:923-927.

18 Pohanka M, Kaňovský P, Bareš M, Pulkrábek J, Rektor I. Pergolide mesylate can improve sexual dysfunction in patients with Parkinson's disease: the result of an open, prospective, 6-month follow-up. *Eur J Neurol* 2004;11:483-488.

19 Klos KJ, Bower JH, Josephs KA, Matsumoto JY, Ahlskog E. Pathological hypersexuality predominately linked to adjuvant dopamine agonist therapy in Parkinson's disease and multiple system atrophy. *Parkinsonism Relat Disord* 2005;11:381-386.

20 Weintraub D, Siderowf AD, Potenza MN, et al. Association of dopamine agonist use with impulse control disorders in Parkinson's disease. *Arch Neurol* 2006;63:969-973.

21 Hussain IF, Brady CM, Swinn MJ, Mathias CJ, Fowler CJ. Treatment of erectile dysfunction with sildenafil citrate (Viagra) in parkinsonism due to Parkinson's disease or multiple system atrophy with observations on orthostatic hypotension. *J Neurol Neurosurg Psychiatry* 2001;71:371-374.

22 Raffaele R, Vecchio I, Giammusso B, Morgia G, Brunetto MB, Rampello L. Efficacy and safety of fixed-dose oral sildenafil in the treatment of sexual dysfunction in depressed patients with idiopathic Parkinson's disease. *Eur Urol* 2002;41:382-386.

23 Cheitlin MD, Hutter AM Jr, Brindis RG, et al. Use of sildenafil (Viagra) in patients with cardiovascular disease. *J Am Coll Cardiol* 1999;33:273-282.

24 Castelli L, Perozzo P, Genesia ML, et al. Sexual well being in parkinsonian patients after deep brain stimulation of the subthalamic nucleus. *J Neurol Neurosurg Psychiatry* 2004;75:1260-1264.

25 Romito LM, Raja M, Daniele A, et al. Transient mania with hypersexuality after surgery for high-frequency stimulation of the subthalamic nucleus in Parkinson's disease. *Mov Disord* 2002;17:1371-1374.

26 Hand A, Gray WK, Chandler BJ, Walker RW. Sexual and relationship dysfunction in people with Parkinson's disease. *Parkinsonism Relat Disord* 2010;16:172-176.

27 Bronner G. Practical strategies for the management of sexual problems in Parkinson's disease. *Parkinsonism Relat Disord* 2009;15(suppl 3):S96-S100.

28 Hartmann U, Burkart M. Erectile dysfunction in patient–physician communication: optimized strategies for addressing sexual issues and the benefit of using a patient questionnaire. *J Sex Med* 2007;4:38-46.

Chapter 10

Gastrointestinal symptoms

Angelo Antonini

Introduction

Gastrointestinal dysfunction is the most common autonomic, non-motor problem in Parkinson's disease (PD), and is more prevalent in patients with PD than in the general population [1–3]. These gastrointestinal disorders, which include salivary excess, dysphagia (difficulty swallowing), nausea/gastroparesis, constipation, and other forms of bowel dysfunction, can cause serious complications, including weight loss [4,5].

Gastrointestinal function is impaired in PD primarily due to disruption to both extrinsic and intrinsic innervation of the gut, partly caused by accumulation of Lewy bodies and neurites in the dorsal motor nucleus of the vagus nerve, sacral parasympathetic nuclei, sympathetic ganglia, and the enteric nervous system [6–9]. All of these regions are involved relatively early in the disease; in fact, constipation may precede motor onset in PD by up to 20 years [10].

Salivary excess

Most patients with PD have excess saliva within the mouth, which often leads to drooling (sialorrhea) [4]. Since the actual production of saliva is in fact decreased in PD, saliva accumulation is caused by poor bolus formation and reduced frequency and efficiency of swallowing [11].

K. R. Chaudhuri et al., *Handbook of Non-Motor Symptoms in Parkinson's Disease*, DOI: 10.1007/978-1-908517-60-9_10,
© Springer Healthcare, a part of Springer Science+Business Media 2011

There are several treatments that can help to lessen excess saliva accumulation. Chewing gum or sucking on hard candy may be useful in social situations [4]. Locally administered anticholinergic drugs work well, although systemically administered agents can produce adverse effects, such as constipation, urinary retention, and cognitive impairment [4,7]. Sublingual atropine ophthalmic drops or ipratropium sprays, as well as botulinum toxin injections into the salivary glands, may decrease saliva production without any systemic adverse effects [4,12].

Dysphagia

It is estimated that anywhere from 30% to over 80% of patients with PD have dysphagia [4,5]. Some believe that dysphagia may occur in the earliest stages of PD [4], while others hypothesize that only late-onset dysphagia is a symptom of PD [13].

The oral, pharyngeal and esophageal stages of swallowing may all be affected in PD. Stiffness, bradykinesia, and possibly tremor of the tongue and oral musculature may slow oral transit time, and residual food may be stuck inside the mouth. Pharyngeal dysmotility can lead to an increased risk of aspiration [4,12].

There is no standard treatment for dysphagia in PD. In some studies, a small minority of patients responded well to dopaminergic medication therapy. Non-pharmacologic methods, including chin-down swallowing, encouraging the patient to eat more slowly, and use of thickened liquids, may be helpful [4,14]. Surgical myotomy or botulinum toxin injection can be conducted if there is no increased risk of aspiration due to the concomitant presence of esophageal dysmotility or lower esophageal sphincter dysfunction with gastroesophageal reflux [4].

Nausea and gastroparesis

In PD, nausea is most often caused by dopaminergic medication therapy. However, it may also develop in patients who are not taking any antiparkinsonian agents. Studies have noted the presence of impaired or delayed gastric emptying (gastroparesis) as the probable etiology for nausea in this population [4,12].

Gastroparesis is present in nearly all patients with PD [15], and appears in even the early stages of the disease [9]. Gastroparesis also may interfere with the efficacy of levodopa, since levodopa must reach the proximal small intestine to be absorbed [9]. This may in turn be the cause of motor response fluctuations in patients receiving levodopa, due to delay in the medication's onset of action or a complete dose failure [4,16].

There are several possible pharmacologic treatment options that may help to accelerate gastric emptying in patients with PD. Domperidone, a dopamine-2-receptor antagonist, has been shown to improve gastric emptying and levodopa absorption, and it does not cross the blood–brain barrier [4,17]. Serotonin 5-HT$_4$ receptor agonists that stimulate acetylcholine release, such as cisapride, tegaserod and mosapride, have prokinetic properties [4]. Cisapride and mosapride both improve gastric emptying in patients with PD [18,19], but use of these drugs has been limited by their cardiotoxicity [4]. Erythromycin, mirtazipine, and botulinum toxin injection are all reported to be effective in improving the gastric emptying process, but have not been formally studied for their use in PD [4].

Bowel dysfunction

Constipation is the most common gastrointestinal problem in patients with PD [4]. In clinical studies, the percentage of patients reporting three or less bowel movements per week ranged from 20% to 89% [4,20]. The severity and rate of occurrence of constipation correlates with disease severity [21,22].

The pathophysiologic basis for reduced bowel movement frequency in PD is decreased colonic smooth muscle and phasic rectal contractions [4,23]. The average colon transit time for patients with PD is more than twice that of people without the disease [23,24]; in one study it was estimated that up to 80% of patients have a prolonged colon transit time [4].

Initial measures to improve bowel movement frequency should include increasing the consumption of fiber and fluids [4]. Patients with PD often have reduced water intake, which leads to constipation [10].

Supplementation with psyllium and other types of fiber fosters bowel movement production in patients with PD [25,26]. A stool softener such as docusate may also be helpful, either given with fiber and fluids or on its own. Other possible medications to alleviate constipation include osmotic laxatives (for short-term use) and prokinetic agents, but dopaminergic agents are not effective [4,27,28].

Difficulty with defecation, resulting in pain, excessive straining, and incomplete elimination, may be present in up to two-thirds of patients with PD [21]. Defecatory dysfunction results when the required muscles do not act in a coordinated fashion, and this may become evident even in early-stage PD [4].

No specific treatment for anorectal dysfunction in PD has been extensively studied. Possible therapies include biofeedback training (to relax the muscles), botulinum toxin injections into the puborectalis muscle, and apomorphine injections [4].

Gastrointestinal effects of PD drugs

Dopamine decreases gastric motility but increases duodenum motility [29]. However, because conversion of levodopa to dopamine in the periphery is usually minimal (due to the concomitant administration of dopamine decarboxylase inhibitors), its use in PD should not have significant effects on gastrointestinal function.

References

1   Greene JG, Noorian AR, Srinivasan S. Delayed gastric emptying and enteric nervous system dysfunction in the rotenone model of Parkinson's disease. *Exp Neurol* 2009;218:154-161.

2   Martinez-Martin P, Schapira AHV, Stocchi F, et al. Prevalence of nonmotor symptoms in Parkinson's disease in an international setting; study using nonmotor symptoms questionnaire in 545 patients. *Mov Disord* 2007;22:1623-1629.

3   Edwards L, Quigley EMM, Hofman R, Pfeiffer RF. Gastrointestinal symptoms in Parkinson's disease: 18-month follow-up study. *Mov Disord* 1993;8:83-86.

4   Pfeiffer RF. Gastrointestinal dysfunction in Parkinson's disease. *Parkinsonism Relat Disord* 2011;17:10-15.

5   Barichella M, Cereda E, Pezzoli G. Major nutritional issues in the management of Parkinson's disease. *Mov Disord* 2009;24:1881-1892.

6   Wakabayashi K, Takahashi H, Ohama E, et al. Lewy bodies in the visceral autonomic nervous system in Parkinson's disease. *Adv Neurol* 1993;60:609-612.

7   Natale G, Pasquali L, Ruggieri S, Paparelli A, Fornai F. Parkinson's disease and the gut: a well known clinical association in need of an effective cure and explanation. *Neurogastroenterol Motil* 2008;20:741-749.

8   Braak H, de Vos RA, Bohl J, Del Tredici K. Gastric α-synuclein immunoreactive inclusions in Meissner's and Auerbach's plexuses in cases staged for Parkinson's disease-related brain pathology. *Neurosci Lett* 2006;396:67-72.

9   Jost WH. Gastrointestinal dysfunction in Parkinson's disease. *J Neurol Sci* 2010;289:69-73.

10 Ueki A, Otsuka M. Life style risks of Parkinson's disease: association between decreased water intake and constipation. *J Neurol* 2004;251(suppl 7):vii/18-23.

11 Nóbrega AC, Rodrigues B, Torres AC, Scarpel RD, Neves CA, Melo A. Is drooling secondary to a swallowing disorder in patients with Parkinson's disease? *Parkinsonism Relat Disord* 2008;14:243-245.

12 Pfeiffer RF. Gastrointestinal, urological, and sexual dysfunction in Parkinson's disease. *Mov Disord* 2010;25(suppl 1):S94-S97.

13 Müller J, Wenning GK, Verny M, et al. Progression of dysarthria and dysphagia in postmortemconfirmed Parkinsonian disorders. *Arch Neurol* 2001;58:259-264.

14 Wood LD, Neumiller JJ, Setter SM, Dobbins EK. Clinical review of treatment options for select nonmotor symptoms of Parkinson's disease. *Am J Geriatr Pharmacother* 2010;8:294-315.

15 Goetze O, Nikodem AB, Wiezcorek J, et al. Predictors of gastric emptying in Parkinson's disease. *Neurogastroenterol Motil* 2006;18:369-375.

16 Hardoff R, Sula M, Tamir A, et al. Gastric emptying time and gastric motility in patients with Parkinson's disease. *Mov Disord* 2001;16:1041-1047.

17 Soykan I, Sarosiek I, Shifflett J, Wooten GF, McCallum W. Effect of chronic oral domperidone therapy on GI symptoms and gastric emptying in patients with Parkinson's disease. *Mov Disord* 1997;12:952-957.

18 Djaldetti R, Koren M, Ziv I, Achiron A, Melamed E. Effect of cisapride on response fluctuations in Parkinson's disease. *Mov Disord* 1995;10:81-84.

19 Asai H, Udaka F, Hirano M, et al. Increased gastric motility during 5-HT$_4$ agonist therapy reduces response fluctuations in Parkinson's disease. *Parkinsonism Relat Disord* 2005;11:499-502.

20 Siddiqui MF, Rast S, Lynn MJ, Auchus AP, Pfeiffer RF. Autonomic dysfunction in Parkinson's disease: a comprehensive symptom survey. *Parkinsonism Relat Disord* 2002;8:277–284.

21 Edwards LL, Pfeiffer RF, Quigley EMM, Hofman R, Balluff M. Gastrointestinal symptoms in Parkinson's disease. *Mov Disord* 1991;6:151-156.

22 Sakakibara R, Shinotoh H, Uchiyama T, et al. Questionnaire-based assessment of pelvic organ dysfunction in Parkinson's disease. *Auton Neurosci* 2001;92:76-85.

23 Sakakibara R, Odaka T, Uchiyama T, et al. Colonic transit time and rectoanal videomanometry in Parkinson's disease. *J Neurol Neurosurg Psychiatry* 2003;74:268-272.

24 Edwards LL, Quigley EMM, Harned RK, Hofman R, Pfeiffer RF. Characterization of swallowing and defecation in Parkinson's disease. *Am J Gastroenterol* 1994;89:15-25.

25 Ashraf W, Pfeiffer RF, Park F, Lof J, Quigley EMM. Constipation in Parkinson's disease: objective assessment and response to psyllium. *Mov Disord* 1997;12:946-951.

26 Astarloa R, Mena MA, Sánchez V, de la Vega L, de Yébenes JG. Clinical and pharmacokinetic effects of a diet rich in insoluble fiber on Parkinson disease. *Clin Neuropharmacol* 1992;15:375-380.

27 Zangaglia R, Martignoni E, Glorioso M, et al. Macrogol for the treatment of constipation in Parkinson's disease. A randomized placebo-controlled study. *Mov Disord* 2007;22:1239-1244.

28 Muzerengi S, Contrafatto D, Chaudhuri KR. Non-motor symptoms: identification and management. *Parkinsonism Relat Disord* 2007;13(suppl 3):S450-S456.

29 Marzio L, Neri M, Pieramico O, Delle Donne M, Peeters TL, Cuccurullo F. Dopamine interrupts GI fed motility pattern in humans. Effect on motilin and somatostatin blood levels. *Dig Dis Sci* 1990;35:327-332.

Chapter 11

Other symptoms

K Ray Chaudhuri

Pain

Parkinson's disease (PD) patients commonly present with severe or intractable pain, which some patients find more distressing than the motor disability [1]. Furthermore, PD-related pain can present in a variety of types (Figure 11.1) and, in up to a quarter of patients, chronic pain precedes the onset of motor symptoms or the start of anti-parkinsonian treatment. However, despite being almost ubiquitous, pain in PD patients often remains poorly managed. In one study, 83% of PD patients reported pain, but only 34% received analgesics [2].

Ascertaining whether pain arises from the pathology underlying PD, co-morbidity or both is often difficult; for example, postural disturbances, rigidity or abnormal movements arising from PD could exacerbate osteoarthritic pain. To complicate matters further, pain categories may overlap; for example, secondary orofacial pain might respond to dopaminergic treatment [3]. Therefore, there is a need to develop validated scales or questionnaires to differentiate and quantify the relative contribution made by PD and co-morbidities to the pain syndrome experienced by a particular patient at any particular time.

Pain associated with PD, rather than co-morbidity, may arise from dysfunctional dopaminergic-dependent centers that regulate autonomic function and inhibit pain [3]. In one study, positron emission tomography

K. R. Chaudhuri et al., *Handbook of Non-Motor Symptoms in Parkinson's Disease*, DOI: 10.1007/978-1-908517-60-9_11, © Springer Healthcare, a part of Springer Science+Business Media 2011

The Chaudhuri–Schapira classification of pain in Parkinson's disease

Musculoskeletal pain	
PD-related chronic pain (may respond to dopaminergic therapy)	Central pain Visceral pain
Fluctuation-related pain (dopaminergic therapy responsive)	Dyskinetic pain Off period dystonia-related pain Off period generalized pain
Nocturnal pain (usually dopaminergic therapy responsive)	Related to restless legs syndrome/periodic limb movement Nocturnal akinesia linked
Coat-hanger pain (rare in PD and linked to postural hypotention)	Temporomandibular joint pain
Orofacial pain	Bruxism-related pain Burning mouth syndrome (may be levodopa responsive)
Peripheral limb/abdominal pain	Drug induced
Pain linked to peripheral edema	
Lower bowel pain related to retroperitoneal fibrosis	

Figure 11.1 The Chaudhuri–Schapira classification of pain in Parkinson's disease. Adapted from Chandhuri & Shapira [2].

(PET) identified over-activation of several nociceptive cerebral areas in response to painful stimuli in PD patients. Levodopa attenuated this over-activation. In parallel, the pain threshold to cold was substantially lower in PD patients who had been withdrawn from anti-parkinsonian treatment compared with controls. Levodopa normalized the threshold [4]. Another study found that PD patients reporting primary central pain showed hyperalgesia, but did not demonstrate habituation of the sympathetic sudomotor response, when exposed to repetitive pain. Again, levodopa improved these abnormalities [5]. However, peripheral mechanisms, such as cramp-like pain related to dystonia, may induce the pain syndrome in some PD patients. Clearly, health-care professionals need to perform detailed and extensive clinical evaluations to optimize care of PD patients with painful non-motor symptoms (NMSs).

Accurately determining the prevalence of pain syndromes among PD patients is problematic. Few epidemiological surveys clearly define 'pain' or enrol a control group. Furthermore, most studies draw patients from tertiary specialized centers and, therefore, the results may not apply to the general PD population.

These caveats notwithstanding, pain is undoubtedly common among PD patients; for example, one study showed 64.9% of 42 female and 54 male PD patients reported pain [1]. Indeed, pain was the first PD symptom to emerge in three patients (2.8%). Musculoskeletal pain was the most frequent presentation, reported by 28 patients (44.4%). Pain secondary to dystonia (19.1%), central pain (12.7%) and radicular or neuropathic pain (11.1%) were also common. Furthermore, 12.7% of PD patients experienced more than one pain type. In this study, pain did not correlate with: sex, PD duration or stage, use of dopamine agonists and levodopa, years of levodopa treatment or current dosage, depression, anxiety or sleep disturbances, age at onset of PD, or history of PD in first-degree relatives [1]. However, people with akathisia were more likely to report pain than those without this movement disorder [1].

Beiske and colleagues [2] found that 83% of 176 home-living PD patients reported pain – a significantly higher proportion than in the general population, based on the SF-36 Bodily Pain Scale. Musculoskeletal pain again emerged as the most common pain type, reported by 70% of patients. Furthermore, 40% of patients reported dystonic pain, 20% radicular or neuropathic pain and 10% central neuropathic pain. Just over half (53%) of patients reported one type of pain, whereas 24% and 5% endured two and three pain types, respectively. Female sex emerged as the only factor associated with pain. Only 34% of patients received analgesics.

Optimizing anti-parkinsonian treatment may alleviate pain associated with motor symptoms, fluctuations and dopamine responsiveness, including 'early morning' or 'off' dystonias, and pseudo-neuropathic syndromes during 'off' periods. Levodopa dose adjustment, alternative treatments (eg, amantadine) or surgery can alleviate exacerbations of osteoarticular pain induced by peak-dose dyskinesias. Evidence is emerging that dopoaminergic therapies may have a beneficial effect on pain. For instance in the recently reported RECOVER study [6,7], the first double-blind placebo controlled trial of rotigotine patch in PD patients reported a significant improvement in pain measured in a likert scale in the PD cases compared to placebo. This result possibly underpins the importance of using longer-acting therapies in PD which may serve to smooth out the motor and non-motor fluctuations in responses, pain being a major aspect of non-motor fluctuation in PD. Further studies need to evaluate the risk–benefit ratios for analgesics across the range of pain syndromes in PD patients. Nevertheless, if modifying dopaminergic treatment fails to alleviate pain adequately or is inappropriate, physicians should consider prescribing analgesics according to the World Health Organization's 'ladder'.

Fatigue

Fatigue in PD may originate from several underlying factors including: central dopaminergic deficit in the limbic area; secondary to other NMSs (eg, sleepiness or orthostatic hypotension); as an adverse event (particularly dopamine agonists); or from co-morbidity [8]. PD patients with fatigue arising from one or more of these causes report profound tiredness, lack of energy or exhaustion, or becoming tired quickly after activity. Apart from reporting worse subjective physical and mental fatigue on self-report questionnaires than controls, PD patients exhibit increased physical fatigability in force generation and finger-tapping tests, and greater mental fatigability. Indeed, PD patients display abnormal performance in all three domains in the attention network test [9].

The pervasive problem posed by fatigue in PD patients commonly leads to reduced activity and markedly impaired quality of life. People with non-fluctuating PD may experience more fatigue and a worse health-related quality of life (HRQoL) compared with patients with diabetes and healthy elderly individuals [10]. Fatigue also impairs HRQoL in non-depressed and non-demented PD patients. Indeed, fatigued patients showed poorer scores on the SF-36 and PDQ-39 emotional well-being, mobility, physical functioning, and social functioning domains compared with unfatigued patients [11].

Although there is little doubt that fatigue is common and distressing for patients, estimates of the prevalence among people with PD vary depending on the definition and assessment method used, the populations tested and the co-morbidities present; for instance, differentiating fatigue from depression secondary to parkinsonism can prove problematic. Nevertheless, Beiske and Svensson [12] estimated that between 37% and 56% of PD patients experience fatigue. A study from Slovakia reported that 81% of 150 PD patients suffered fatigue. Physical fatigue emerged as a particular problem, and mood disorders and Unified Parkinson's Disease Rating Scale (UPDRS) scores both predicted the severity of fatigue [13].

Optimization of pharmacotherapy may alleviate fatigue in some patients. Levodopa and modafinil reduce physical fatigability, methylphenidate can alleviate subjective fatigue and psychostimulants improve mental fatigue. A recent study using positron emission tomography (PET) has shown that fatigue may be associated with a specific sertonergic deficit in the striatal and thalamic areas in PD suggesting that tthere may be a possible role of serotonergic therapies for treatment of fatigue in future [14]. Interestingly, the RECOVER study also reported a significant beneficial effect of the rotigotine patch on fatigue as judged by the NMSS sub-item score compared to placebo [15]. Development of gold standard methods to measure fatigue in patients with PD is still an unmet need as is specific treatments for this common and debilitating NMS [9].

Weight changes

Weight loss can emerge before motor symptoms [16]; for example, Lewy bodies in the myenteric plexus can cause constipation, which may predate the diagnosis of PD by many years. Nevertheless, the differential diagnosis should exclude co-morbid conditions, such as thyrotoxicosis, depression, tuberculosis or other cryptic infection, and neoplasia. PD patients showing an acute onset or worsening of dysphagia or constipation with concurrent weight loss, iron deficiency anemia or rectal bleeding should undergo prompt gastrointestinal investigation.

Several factors interact to influence body weight among PD patients, although the relative importance of each remains controversial [17]. Increased metabolism or physical activity does not fully account for weight loss in many PD patients. Changes in appetite, the pathogenesis of which is unknown, probably also contribute [16]. Untreated and suboptimally treated PD patients seem to exhibit increased resting energy expenditure, partly due to rigidity and dyskinesias [17].

As PD advances, many patients progressively lose weight due to poor nutrition. Nevertheless, the decline in fat mass often begins several years before diagnosis, despite the tendency of many patients with early PD to increase energy intake. The decline worsens as PD progresses, exacerbated by poor motor control and suboptimal treatment [17]; for instance, chronic levodopa treatment may induce hypersecretion of insulin and · growth hormone, which may trigger lipolysis and, therefore, increase basal metabolic rate [17]. Finally, reduced energy intake may also contribute to weight loss in PD patients. Motor symptoms potentially restrict activities of daily living, including cooking or shopping. Malabsorption, olfactory dysfunction, dysphagia and impaired cognition can further impede feeding [18] and exacerbate weight loss.

As weight loss increases the risk of infection and decubitus ulcers, as well as exacerbating motor, behavioral and autonomic impairment [18], health-care professionals should measure weight at each clinical review. On the other hand, some PD patients gain weight, again for a variety of reasons. Pallidotomy and deep brain stimulation can produce significant weight gain, possibly due to symptomatic improvement, reduction in levodopa-induced dyskinesias, and attenuation of insulin and growth hormone hypersecretion. Dopamine agonists may also produce weight gain, possibly by stimulating compulsive eating or alleviating depression. Finally, weight gain may also emerge from abnormal neuroendocrine regulation, such as dysfunctional corticotrophin-releasing hormone and orexin-related signalling pathways [17].

Future studies need to elucidate many of the molecular details underlying weight change in PD and characterize the optimal treatment. In the meantime, physicians should consider four principles when managing patients. First, dietitians should develop a nutritional balance that prevents body weight changes. Second, physicians should optimize levodopa pharmacokinetics by avoiding drug–diet interaction with proteins and other nutrients. Third, physicians should actively manage gastrointestinal dysfunction, including dysphagia, gastro-oesophageal reflux and constipation. Finally, the multidisciplinary team should remain cognisant of the importance of preventing, detecting and treating nutritional deficiencies, especially those affecting micronutrients and vitamins [17].

In conclusion, sensory disorders, fatigue and weight changes are among the most common NMSs experienced by PD patients, can offer a marker of early disease and appear to be associated with a poor prognosis. Yet these NMSs remain under-reported, under-recognized and poorly understood. Furthermore, therapeutic nihilism hinders optimal management. Future studies need to develop improved instruments to detect and follow these NMSs as well as characterize evidence-based treatments to improve HRQoL, function outcomes and prognosis for PD patients with these common causes of discomfort, distress and disability.

References

1   Hanagasi HA, Akat S, Gurvit H, et al. Pain is common in Parkinson's disease. *Clin Neurol Neurosurg* 2010;113:11-13.

2   Beiske AG, Loge JH, Ronningen A, Svensson E. Pain in Parkinson's disease: Prevalence and characteristics. *Pain* 2009;141;173-177.

3   Chaudhuri K, Schapira A. Non-motor symptoms of Parkinson's disease: dopaminergic pathophysiology and treatment. *Lancet Neurol* 2009;8:464-474.

4   Brefel-Courbon C, Payoux P, Thalamas C, et al. Effect of levodopa on pain threshold in Parkinson's disease: a clinical and positron emission tomography study. *Mov Disord* 2005;20:1557-1563.

5   Schestatsky P, Kumru H, Valls-Sole J, et al. Neurophysiologic study of central pain in patients with Parkinson disease. *Neurology* 2007;69:2162-2169.

6   Trenkwalder C, Kies B, Rudzinska M, et al; and the RECOVER study group. Rotigotine effects on early morning motor function and sleep in Parkinson's disease: A double-blind, randomised, placebo-controlled study (RECOVER). *Mov Disord* 2011;26:90-99.

7   Kassubek J, Ghys L, Chaudhuri KR, et al; on behalf of the RECOVER study investigators. Transdermal rotigotine improves pain in patients with Parkinson's disease: a post hoc analysis of the RECOVER Study. Poster presented at: Deutschen Gesellschaft für Neurologie (DGN), 84th Annual Congress; September 28-October 1, 2011; Wiesbaden, Germany.

8   Park A, Stacy M. Non-motor symptoms in Parkinson's disease. J Neurol 2009;256:293-298.

9   Lou JS. Physical and mental fatigue in Parkinson's disease: epidemiology, pathophysiology and treatment. *Drugs Aging* 2009;26:195-208.

10   Larsen JP, Karlsen K, Tandberg E. Clinical problems in non-fluctuating patients with Parkinson's disease: A community based study. *Mov Disord* 2000;15:826-829.

11   Herlofson K and Larsen JP. The influence of fatigue on health-related quality of life in patients with Parkinson's disease. *Acta Neurol Scand* 2003;107:1-6.

12   Beiske AG, Svensson E. Fatigue in Parkinson's disease: a short update. *Acta Neurol Scand Suppl* 2010;190:78-81.

13   Havlikova E, Rosenberger J, Nagyova I, et al. Clinical and psychosocial factors associated with fatigue in patients with Parkinson's disease. *Parkinsonism Relat Disord* 2008;14:187-192.

14   Pavese N, Metta V, Bose SK, et al. Fatigue in Parkinson's disease is linked to striatal and limbic serotonergic dysfunction. *Brain* 2010;133:3434-3443.

15   Chaudhuri KR, Friedman JH, Surmann E, et al; on behalf of the RECOVER study investigators. The effects of transdermal rotigotine on mood/cognition: interpretations from a post hoc analysis of the RECOVER Study using the Parkinson's disease Non-Motor Symptom Scale. Poster presented at: 15th International Congress of Parkinson's Disease and Movement Disorders; June 5-9, 2011; Toronto, Canada.

16   Korczyn AD, Gurevich T. Parkinson's disease: before the motor symptoms and beyond. *J Neurol Sci* 2010;289:2-6.

17   Barichella M, Cereda E, Pezzoli G. Major nutritional issues in the management of Parkinson's disease. *Mov Disord* 2009;24:1881-1892.

18   Kashihara K. Weight loss in Parkinson's disease. *J Neurol* 2006;253(suppl 7):VII38-VII41.